RENAL DIET COOKBOOK

FOR BEGINNERS

YOU DON'T NEED

1500 RECIPES

TO IMPROVE YOUR KIDNEYS AND REGAIN STRENGTH

DISCOVER MORE THAN 250 ENERGY-BOOSTING RECIPES, LOW ON POTASSIUM, PHOSPHORUS AND SODIUM, AND ENJOY THE TASTE OF SALT AGAIN!

By Susan Meadow

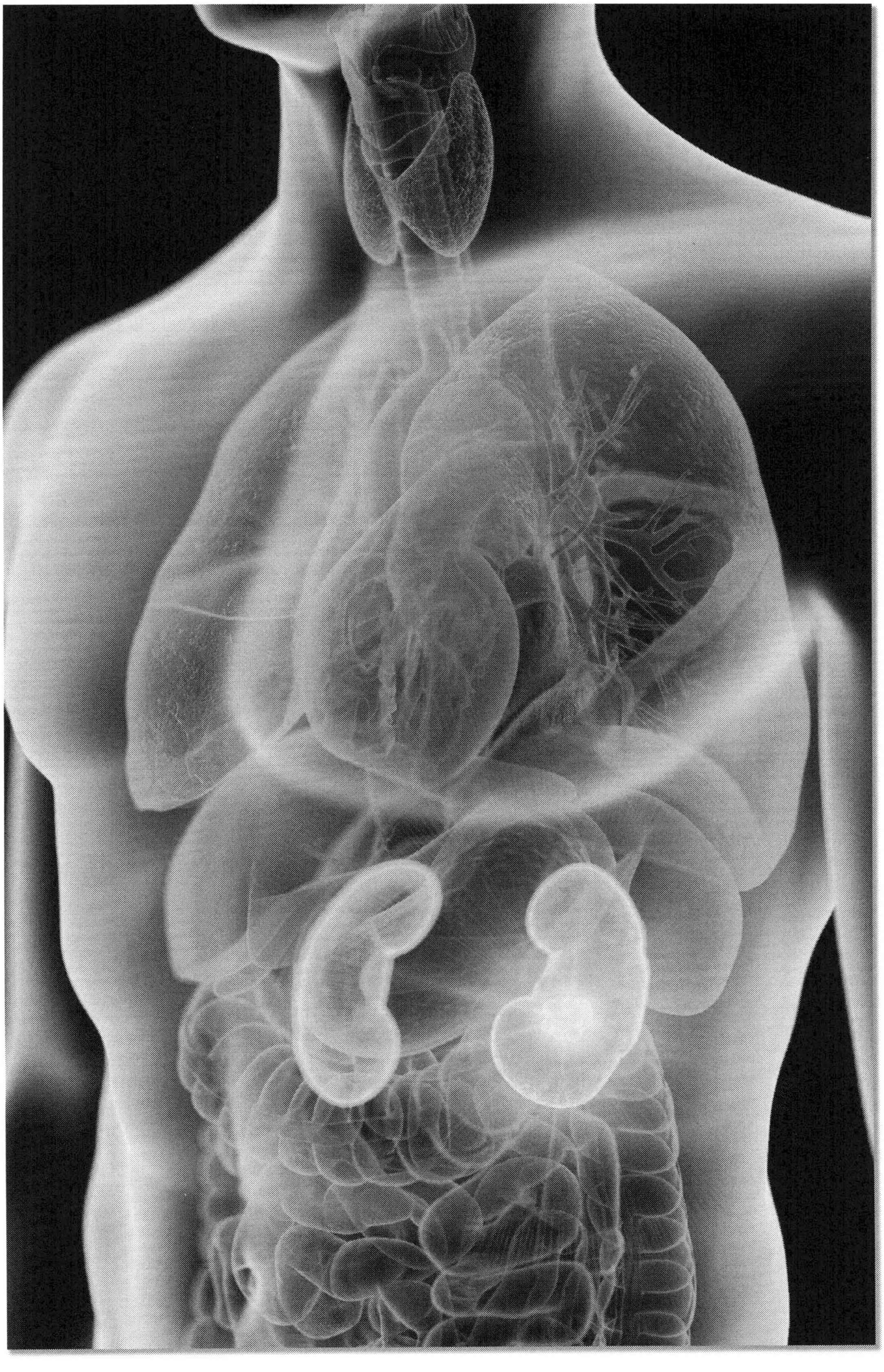

© Copyright 2022-2023 - All rights reserved.

The content contained within this book may not be reproduced, duplicated, or transmitted without direct written permission from the author or the publisher.

Under no circumstances will any blame or legal responsibility be held against the publisher, or author, for any damages, reparation, or monetary loss due to the information contained within this book. Either directly or indirectly.

Legal Notice:

This book is copyright protected. This book is only for personal use. You cannot amend, distribute, sell, use, quote or paraphrase any part, or the content within this book, without the consent of the author or publisher.

Disclaimer Notice:

Please note the information contained within this document is for educational and entertainment purposes only. All effort has been executed to present accurate, up to date, and reliable, complete information. No warranties of any kind are declared or implied. Readers acknowledge that the author is not engaging in the rendering of medical or professional advice. The content within this book has been derived from various sources. Please consult a licensed professional before attempting any techniques outlined in this book.

By reading this document, the reader agrees that under no circumstances is the author responsible for any losses, direct or indirect, which are incurred as a result of the use of information contained within this document, including, but not limited to, — errors, omissions, or inaccuracies

TABLE OF CONTENTS

INTRODUCTION 1
- The Renal Diet: How Does It Work, and Benefits 4
- Understand Your Nutrients Needs 6
- How To Reduce Your Phosphorus Intake? 8
- How To Monitor Your Potassium Levels? 10
- How To Decrease Your Sodium Intake? 14
- Reasons Why You Should Monitor Your Sodium Intake 15
- How To Monitor Your Sodium Intake? 15

FOOD THAT YOU MUST AVOID 16
- Foods to Eat 17
- Fluids and Juices for Healthy Kidneys 18

SHOPPING LIST, AND MEAL PLAN 19
- Renal Diet Shopping List 20

MEAL PLAN 26
- Week 1 Meal Plan 27
- Week 2 Meal Plan 27
- Week 3 Meal Plan 28
- Week 4 Meal Plan 28

DIETARY STAGES OF RENAL DIET 29
- Stage one 30
- Stage two 30
- Stage three 30
- Stage four 31
- Stage five 31

BREAKFAST 33
- Peach Berry Parfait 34
- Open-Faced Bagel Breakfast Sandwich 34
- Bulgur Bowl with Strawberries and Walnuts 35
- Overnight Oats Three Ways 35
- Buckwheat Pancakes 36
- Apple and Cinnamon French Toast Strata 37
- Broccoli Basil Quiche 37
- Asparagus Frittata 38
- Poached Eggs with Cilantro Butter 39
- Green Breakfast Soup 39
- Tasty Pancakes 40
- Slow Cooked Oats 40
- Papaya Orange Smoothie 41
- Brown Muffins 41
- Easy Corn Pudding 42
- Sliced Apple Cookies 43
- Chocolate Muffins 43
- Savory Spring Muffins 44
- Pita with Egg & Curry 44

HOT VANILLA CEREALS	45
AROMATIC CARROT CREAM	46
MUSHROOMS VELVET SOUP	47
EASY LETTUCE WRAPS	48
SPAGHETTI WITH PESTO	49
SPICED WRAPS	49
POACHED ASPARAGUS AND EGG	50
APPLE TURNOVER	50
EGG DROP SOUP	51
ROASTED PEPPER SOUP	51
ASSORTED FRESH FRUIT JUICE	52
RASPBERRY AND PINEAPPLE SMOOTHIE	53
MEXICAN FRITTATA	53
OLIVE OIL AND SESAME ASPARAGUS	54
BREAKFAST CHEESECAKE	54
EGGS CREAMY MELT	55
STUFFED CRIMINI MUSHROOMS WITH BASIL PESTO	55
DILLY SCRAMBLED EGGS WITH GOAT CHEESE	56
REDUCED-FAT BREAKFAST CASSEROLE	56
BREAKFAST CEREAL MIX	57
FRENCH TOAST WITH TASTY STRAWBERRY CREAM CHEESE	57
CREAM CHEESE GOLDEN BAGEL	58
JAZZ APPLE OATMEAL	58
QUICK AND EASY COFFEE CUP EGG SCRAMBLE	59
PEPPERS AND ONIONS SCRAMBLED EGG WRAP	59
REFRESHING AND TASTY SMOOTHIE	60
PROTEIN-PACKED TOFU SCRABLER	60
60-SECONDS OMELETS WITH VEGGIES	61
SAUSAGE BREAKFAST MUFFIN WITH EGG AND CHEESE	61
HIGH-PROTEIN PEACH SMOOTHIE	62
TASTY BREAKFAST TORTILLAS WITH RED HOT JALAPENO	62
BREAKFAST BAR WITH BRAN AND OATMEAL	63
SWEET CREPES WITH APPLES	63
SWEET AND CRUNCHY POPCORN	64
FIBER BOOSTER BARS	65
CRANBERRY OATMEAL AND VANILLA COOKIES	65
CHOCOLATE BANANA OATMEAL MORNING-BOOST	66
EGG AND SAUSAGE BRUNCH	66
STUFFED ANAHEIM CHILI PEPPERS	67
PUFFED TORTILLAS BREAKFAST	68
TASTY VEGAN BREAKFAST	69
LUNCH	**71**
SALAD WITH VINAIGRETTE	72
SALAD WITH LEMON DRESSING	72
SHRIMP WITH SALSA	73
CAULIFLOWER SOUP	74
CABBAGE STEW	74
RICE AND CHICKEN SOUP	75
HERBED CHICKEN	76
PESTO PORK CHOPS	77
VEGETABLE CURRY	77
GRILLED STEAK WITH SALSA	78

- Eggplant and Red Pepper Soup ... 79
- Persian Chicken ... 80
- Pork Souvlaki ... 80
- Chicken Stew ... 81
- Baked Flounder ... 81
- Caraway Cabbage and Rice ... 82
- Chicken and Sweet Potato Stir Fry ... 82
- Chicken and Asparagus Pasta ... 83
- Hawaiian Rice ... 84
- Shrimp Fried Rice ... 84
- Vegetarian Egg Fried Rice ... 85
- Autumn Orzo Salad ... 86
- Blackened Shrimp and Pineapple Salad ... 86
- Green Pepper Slaw ... 87
- Cranberries and Couscous Salad ... 87
- Tuna Salad ... 88
- Roasted Vegetable Salad ... 88
- Chicken Pita Pizza ... 89
- Chicken Wraps ... 90
- Mexican Chicken Pizza ... 90
- Energetic Fruity Salad ... 91
- Appealing Green Salad ... 91
- Excellent Veggie Sandwiches ... 92
- Lunchtime Staple Sandwiches ... 92
- Greek Style Pita Rolls ... 93
- Healthier Pita Veggie Rolls ... 93
- Crunchy Veggie Wraps ... 94
- Surprisingly Tasty Chicken Wraps ... 94
- Authentic Shrimp Wraps ... 95
- Loveable Tortillas ... 95
- Elegant Veggie Tortillas ... 96
- Delightful Pizza ... 96
- Winner Kabobs ... 97
- Tempting Burgers ... 97
- Tastiest Meatballs ... 98

DINNER ... 100

- Lemon Sprouts ... 101
- Lemon and Broccoli Platter ... 101
- Chicken Liver Stew ... 102
- Mushroom Cream Soup ... 102
- Garlic Soup ... 103
- Simple Lamb Chops ... 103
- Garlic and Butter-Flavored Cod ... 104
- Tilapia Broccoli Platter ... 104
- Parsley Scallops ... 105
- Blackened Chicken ... 105
- Spicy Paprika Lamb Chops ... 106
- Steamed Fish ... 106
- Mushroom and Olive Sirloin Steak ... 107
- Kale and Garlic Platter ... 107
- Blistered Beans and Almond ... 108
- Eggplant Crunchy Fries ... 108

Oregano Salmon with Crunchy Crust 109
Broiled Shrimp 109
Shrimp Spaghetti 110
Teriyaki Tuna 110
Chicken Noodle Soup 111
Beef Stew with Apple Cider 111
Chicken Chili 112
Tofu Stir Fry 112
Broccoli Pancake 113
Tangy Whole Roasted Sea Bass with Oregano 113
Pan-Seared Salmon Salad with Lemon-Dressing 114
Grilled Steak served with Creamy Peanut Sauce 114
Lean Steak with Oregano-Lemon Chimichurri & Arugula Salad 115
Herbed London Broil 116
Ground Beef Tacos 116
Pepper Crusted Steak 117
Stir-Fried Chicken with Water Chestnuts 117
Lemon Garlic Salmon 118
Pan-Fried Chili Beef with Toasted Cashews 118
Healthy Keto Coconut-Lime Skirt Steak 119
Spicy Grilled Cod 120
Healthy Low-Carb Grilled Turkey 120
Satisfying Arugula Salad with Fruit & Chicken 121
Tasty Coconut Cod 121

SIDES AND SNACKS 123

Citrus Sesame Cookies 124
Traditional Spritz Cookies 124
Classic Baking Powder Biscuits 125
Crunchy Chicken Salad Wraps 125
Tasty Chicken Meatballs 126
Herb Roasted Cauliflower 126
Sauteed Butternut Squash 127
German Braised Cabbage 127
Walnut Pilaf 128
Wild Mushroom Couscous 128
Spicy Kale Chips 129
Cinnamon Tortilla Chips 129
Sweet and Spicy Kettle Corn 130
Five-Spice Chicken Lettuce Wraps 130
Meringue Cookies 131
Cornbread 131
Roasted Red Pepper and Chicken Crostini 132
Baba Ghanoush 132
Mixed-Grain Hot Cereal 133
Cinnamon-Nutmeg Blueberry Muffins 133
Fruit and Cheese Breakfast Wrap 134
Egg-In-The-Hole 134
Skillet-Baked Pancake 135
Tuna Cucumber Bites 135
Cinnamon Candied Almonds 136

FISH AND SEAFOODS ENTRÉES..138

    GRILLED SHRIMP WITH CUCUMBER LIME SALSA..139
    SHRIMP SCAMPI LINGUINE...139
    CRAB CAKES WITH LIME SALSA..140
    SEAFOOD CASSEROLE..141
    SWEET GLAZED SALMON..141
    HERB-CRUSTED BAKED HADDOCK...142
    SHORE LUNCH–STYLE SOLE..142
    BAKED COD WITH CUCUMBER-DILL SALSA...143
    CILANTRO-LIME FLOUNDER..144
    HERB PESTO TUNA..144
    GRILLED CALAMARI WITH LEMON AND HERBS...145
    LEMONY HADDOCK...145
    GLAZED SALMON..146
    TUNA CASSEROLE...146
    OREGANO SALMON WITH CRUNCHY CRUST..147
    SARDINE FISH CAKES..147
    CAJUN CATFISH...148
    POACHED GENNARO/SEABASS WITH RED PEPPERS...148
    4-INGREDIENTS SALMON FILLET...149
    OREGANO GRILLED CALAMARI...149
    BAKED SHRIMP CRABS..150
    SALMON STUFFED PASTA..150

MEAT AND POULTRY ENTRÉES...152

    BAKED PORK CHOPS...153
    BEEF KABOBS WITH PEPPER...153
    CABBAGE AND BEEF FRY...154
    MUSHROOM AND OLIVE SIRLOIN STEAK..154
    CALIFORNIA PORK CHOPS...155
    BEEF CHORIZO..155
    PORK FAJITAS..156
    CARIBBEAN TURKEY CURRY..156
    CHICKEN FAJITAS...157
    CHICKEN VERONIQUE...158
    LONDON BROIL...158
    SIRLOIN WITH SQUASH AND PINEAPPLE..159
    SLOW-COOKED BBQ BEEF..159
    BARLEY CHICKEN SALAD...160
    CHICKEN COLESLAW SALAD...160
    BERRY-CHICKEN PASTA SALAD...161
    MEXICAN-STYLE CHICKEN SALAD..162
    SATAY-INSPIRED CHICKEN SALAD..162
    GRILLED CHIMICHURRI CHICKEN KEBABS..163
    ROASTED HERB AND LEMON CHICKEN WITH MASHED SWEET POTATOES...................................164
    CHICKEN AND BROCCOLI PAN BAKE..164
    MOROCCAN CHICKEN AND VEGETABLE STEW...165
    MUSHROOM TURKEY BURGERS WITH POWERHOUSE SALSA...166
    THAI-STYLE CHICKEN STIR-FRY...166
    VEGETABLE AND TURKEY KEBABS..167
    TURKEY PHO..167
    TURKEY-ASPARAGUS RISOTTO..168
    TURKEY TENDERLOIN WITH BERRY SAUCE...169

DESSERTS 171

- Dessert Cocktail 172
- Baked Egg Custard 172
- Gumdrop Cookies 173
- Apple Crunch Pie 173
- Spiced Peaches 174
- Vanilla Custard 174
- Blueberry and Apple Crisp 175
- Lemon Mousse 175
- Raspberry Popsicle 176
- Easy Fudge 176
- Hearty Cucumber Bites 177
- Cauliflower Bagel 177
- Almond Crackers 178
- Cashew and Almond Butter 178
- Nut and Chia Mix 179
- Very Berry Bread Pudding 179
- Sunburst Lemon Bars 180
- Creamy Mint Chocolate Brownies 181
- Festive Cream Cheese Sugar Cookies 181
- Dandelion Green Smoothie 182
- Chocolate Chip Cookies 182
- Baked Peaches with Cream Cheese 183
- Strawberry Ice Cream 183
- Raspberry Brûlée 184

SAUCES, DRESSING AND SEASONINGS 186

- Easy Garlicky Cherry Tomato Sauce 187
- Roasted Onion Dip 187
- Golden Turmeric Sauce 188
- Creamy Turmeric Dressing 189
- Dijon Mustard Vinaigrette 189
- Anti-Inflammatory Caesar Dressing 190
- Fresh Tomato Vinaigrette 190
- Ginger Sesame Sauce 191
- Golden Turmeric Tahini Sauce 191
- Healthy Teriyaki Sauce 192
- Yogurt Garlic Sauce 192
- Chunky Tomato Sauce 193
- Sweet Balsamic Dressing 193
- Citrus Salad Sauce 194
- Anti-Inflammatory Applesauce 194
- Dried Herb Rub 195
- Mediterranean Seasoning 195
- Hot Curry Powder 196
- Cajun Seasoning 196
- Ras El Hanout 197
- Poultry Seasoning 197
- Adobo Seasoning Mix 198
- Herbs De Provence 198
- Honey Mustard 199
- Pickles 199
- Teriyaki Sauce 200

Alfredo Sauce	200
Tomato Salsa	201
Fajita Flavor Marinade	201
Garlic-Herb Seasoning	202
Lime Caribbean Dressing	202

BONUS CHAPTER: 204

WORKOUT FOR KIDNEY PATIENTS: 204

KEEPING ACTIVE DESPITE KIDNEY DISEASE 204

EXERCISES TO INCREASE FLEXIBILITY* 206

    SHOULDER ROTATION 208
    chest and upper back stretch 209
    Leg Stretches 210

AEROBIC EXERCISES* 211

STRENGTH EXERCISES* 213

    Bicep curl: 214
    Leg Lift 215

TIPS AND PRECAUTIONS TO BE CONSIDERED WHEN EXERCISING FOR KIDNEY HEALTH PROBLEMS ...216

CONCLUSION 217

CONVERSION TABLES 219

SHOPPING RESOURCES 224

    Things to Avoid on a Renal Diet 231

REFERENCES 233

RECIPE INDEX 234

INTRODUCTION

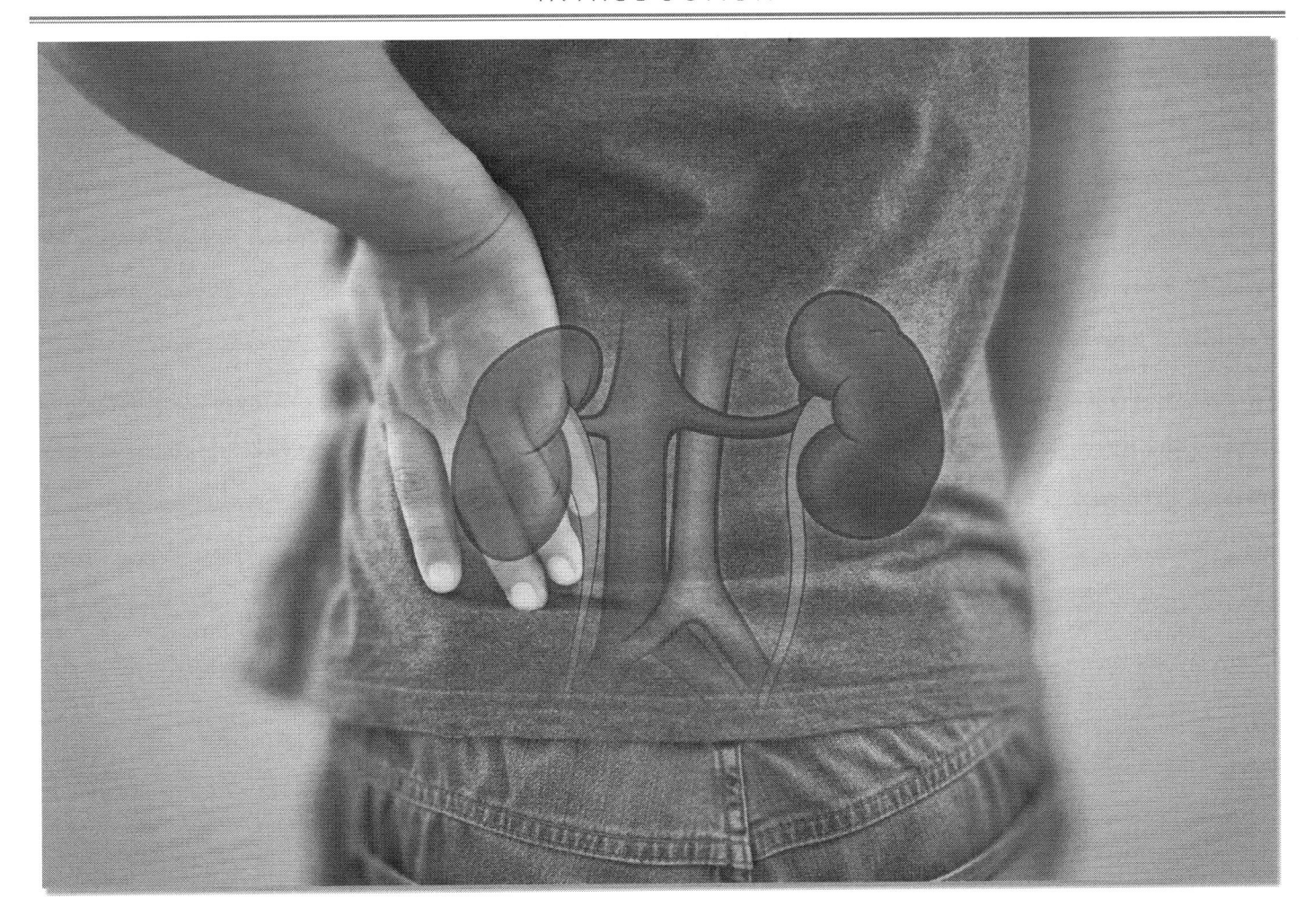

Kidney disease is a medical condition in which one or both of the kidneys fail to perform their proper function. This is the ultimate cause of many problems that put a person's health in serious jeopardy. The disease is progressive and at times, can prove almost fatal.

A dietician recommends a person suffering from this disease should follow a special diet plan.

The plan not only helps treat the condition but also has additional health benefits. This diet helps minimize the side effects of the drugs used to treat the disease and also treats other medical conditions that have a strong link with an unhealthy kidney.

Kidney disease is a serious medical condition. Often, severe symptoms start showing in the early stages of the condition. It is not uncommon to have health experts overlook kidney problems unless the problem is more severe.

Unfortunately, only when the symptoms become severe that the disease becomes impossible to ignore. The good news is that although the disease is serious, it can be treated in most cases. Treatment is done with medications, strict monitoring, diet and lifestyle changes.

The treatment for kidney disease has a lot more benefits than just treating the condition. High cholesterol, high blood pressure, diabetes, overweight, heart disease and other related condition are directly linked to kidney disease. In such a case, treating kidney disease alone not only treats the condition but also minimizes the chances of developing other related health problems in the future.

On the other hand, treating only the symptoms means more drugs and more tests. This can turn out to be very costly but does not address the root cause of a health problem.

Kidneys are major organs that are present in the human body. These two small organs are vital to the body for the removal of harmful waste products from the body. The kidneys also play an important role in releasing the acids, salts and other chemicals required for maintaining the right pH levels of the body tissue. The health of the kidneys is critical to our overall health.

Any disease or malfunctioning of these organs can lead to serious health issues. It is this reason that someone suffering from the disease should be very careful about their diet and lifestyle choices.

A renal diet is a special diet that helps treat and prevent kidney disorders. A person with kidney disease should follow such diet strictly for a prolonged period of time. The diet not only treats the primary disorder but also has additional advantages for maintaining a better health.

Most people know that renal diet is only for people with kidney problems but what they are not aware of is the fact that some dietary changes can help treat other health conditions.

The diet is simple, and the changes are made easy by using readymade substitutes. These alternatives taste like the original and bring in the necessary nutritional value.

Drinking enough water is necessary. The body should be given enough water to flush out the toxins from the body. Even during treatment, drinking water helps keep the kidneys working efficiently. The need for drinking water is even more for someone suffering from kidney disease. A person with a kidney disorder needs to drink water on a regular basis.

Changing the daily routine and lifestyle of a person is very important. The Renal diet recommends the avoidance of certain foods and drinks. People suffering from kidney disease have to avoid certain meals or foods.

These changes can be difficult for people who are used to consuming these items. It is important to note that the changes have to be made for the treatment to be effective. A doctor's advice is very important, and in some cases, it is mandatory to avoid certain foods or beverages.

One important aspect of a renal diet is to check the ingredients of food products. Many food items in the market are complicated with harmful additives and harmful chemicals.

It is recommended that such food products are made a part of a regular diet. Food items that are made in additive-free conditions should be preferred.

Reading the labels of the food package is a good idea. It is very important to avoid sweetened drinks, candied fruits, and sugary foods. Sugars and refined salts should be avoided to a great extent. It is important to consume foods rich in fiber. Lean meat, skinless poultry, fish, fresh fruits, vegetables, and whole grains contribute to a healthy diet. The diet should be supplemented with plenty of liquids. Healthcare experts recommend drinking more fluids in addition to water.

There are different levels of food restrictions. The general rule to follow is to avoid all forms of sugar and foods with simple carbohydrates. It is important to maintain a healthy diet and follow the instructions of the doctor. A healthy diet is not only good for a healthy life but also for the overall functioning of the kidneys. In addition, following the diet prescribed by the renal diet can help treat other health disorders.

Ways to follow Renal diet

There are three special food groups that are involved when it comes to the renal diet. These food groups include:

1. Avoid foods that are high on fat, especially saturated fats...
2. There is the consideration of protein sources, especially those that may be low in fat...
3. There is also the consideration of fruits and vegetables...

In addition to the three food groups above, it is important to consider these three facts:

First, following a renal diet means you can't have certain foods and beverages. The first restriction is beverages that have sugar.

Second, it should be noted that a renal diet is low in salt. Table salt should be avoided at all costs. If table salt is used, it should be in small amounts. This means that seasoning for food must be homemade or purchased at a grocery store that has natural seasonings. They include herbs and spices.

Third, you should know that a renal diet is restricted to foods that have a lot of protein. This is especially important when a person has diabetes. A diet should not have more than two or three servings per week of protein. This includes poultry. Meat, fish and eggs. These foods should be reduced to one serving per week. Some of these foods are mentioned under the following classifications of food.

The other food restriction has to do with fruit. First, it is important to remember that a renal diet is restricted to certain fruits. These fruits are citrus fruit with the skin on. These include oranges, lemons, limes, grapefruits, and tangerines. The second food restriction involves sugars that are in fruit juices. These juices should be avoided. Instead of juice, water should be used to wash down the food.

There are certain vegetables that are also restricted. These include celery, beets, chard, spinach, parsnips, and Brussels sprouts. Legumes, beans, and dry peas are also restricted.

The renal diet is different for every individual. It is important for every person to follow their recommendations and guidelines.

THE RENAL DIET: HOW DOES IT WORK, AND BENEFITS

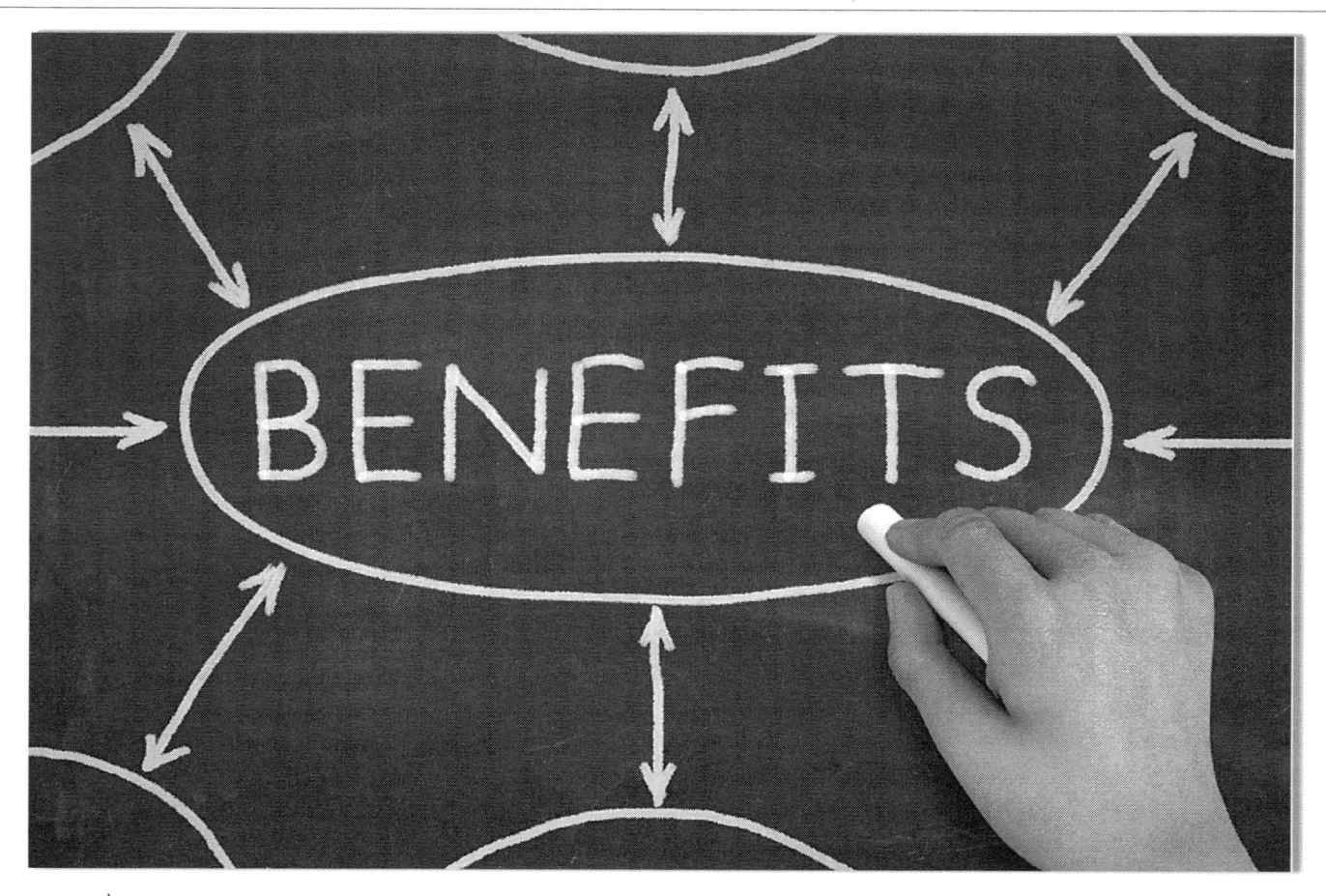

Renal diet refers to a diet that focuses on making sure your kidneys are taken care of. You should avoid protein products that will ultimately worsen the kidneys and even cause long term damages to your health.

A renal diet is very important for people who are either suffering from kidney disease or patients who suffer from previous disorders of their kidneys, a renal diet focuses on the intake of different types of foods that can only beneficially impact the body's health.

The renal diet also focuses on the amount of food intake you should take daily to make sure you maintain a good amount of nutrition and also do not eat too much that can worsen the condition of your kidney.

How Does It Work?

The renal diet focuses on making sure you get a good amount of nutrients without; you know actually eating too much protein. Protein in a normal diet is usually necessary for the health, but sometimes it can worsen the conditions of kidneys too much. Usually, renal diets restrict the amount of protein intake to the minimum amount necessary for the body and the rest of the nutrients should be supplied.

This is the main idea of the renal diet, as to how your kidneys absorb the different nutrients because everyone is different. If you are suffering from a previous renal illness or disease, you likely will not be able to handle the same amount of protein as benefits someone else. Also, you need to make sure that you will stick to this diet strictly to ensure the best results.

Benefits of Renal Diet:

The renal diet is designed for patients with previous renal disease and also those who suffer from people with renal disease. The diet is a specialized version of other general diet and is known to improve the clinical conditions and function of the patient. It does so by reducing the risk of complications and minimizing the damage from vascular injury of the kidneys. The diet has shown to improve the survival rate of the patient, reduce the risk for dialysis and can even consist of reduced medications. By eating the right food in the right amount, it is known to improve the function of the patient and also minimize the damage to the body.

The diet so far is known to have a lot of benefits for the body. Many experts have recommended this diet because of the health benefits it can have. The diet improves the survival rate of the patient, reduces the risk of dialysis, and even reduces the risk for complications. The diet can even help in reducing the number of medications needed for those who suffer from kidney problems. That being said, there are certain things that are really to consider before following a renal diet. This is usually accompanied by a doctor or other health care provider. The benefits of the diet are well established and the fact that the diet improves your health in the long term.

The diet is known to be a restrictive diet, but it is not restricted to a person depending on the condition of their kidney. In fact, the diet is designed for those who have already suffered from damage to their kidney. A renal diet is recommended by experts in the field to improve the overall health of the patient.

The diet is known to enforce other clinical recommendations and the diet, helps to improve the functions of the kidneys. A renal diet has many restrictions on what you can eat but it is important to actually stick to the diet to prevent any further damage to the body. Also, remember you may need to get your diet approved by your doctor, to ensure that you are following the diet properly.

The renal diet is a special diet that focuses on improving the health of the patient and can be beneficial if the patient suffers from renal disease. To ensure that you have the best of the diet, make sure you stick to the diet advice given by your doctor.

UNDERSTAND YOUR NUTRIENTS NEEDS

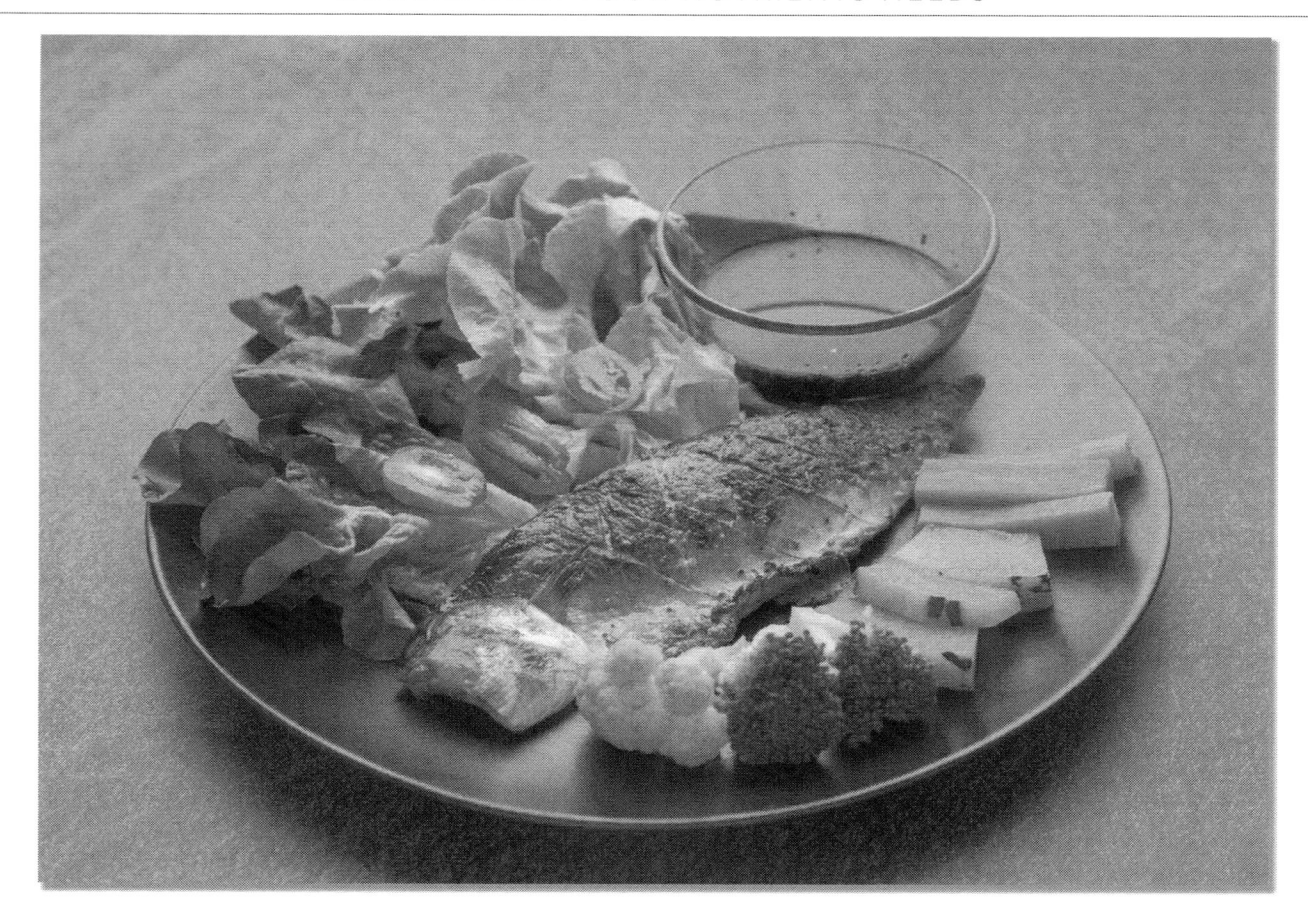

Changing your food and lifestyle can help you manage your kidney disease and stop it from progressing to more serious stages. If you have kidney disease, you should become familiar with the following food and nutrient groups.

Carbohydrates: Since they are your body's main source of energy, carbohydrates should make up the bulk of your diet. The two different forms of carbohydrates are complex and simple. Fruit is an illustration of a simple carbohydrate. Fruit is packed with the fiber, vitamins, and energy that your body needs. Examples of complex carbohydrates are grains, bread, and vegetables. All these carbohydrates provide minerals and vitamins as well as energy and fiber. Carbohydrates also play a vital role in balancing blood sugar levels.

Proteins: They are directly involved in the chemical processes essential for life, and are your body's disease-fighting mechanisms. They repair tissue and build muscle. These are your body's defense against disease. Animal foods are the primary sources of protein, such as milk, beef, eggs, chicken, and pork. Protein can also be found in some plants. Legumes, nuts, and soybean products are all good sources of proteins. Vegetables also contain small amounts of protein. However, as chronic kidney disease progresses, your renal dietitian may recommend you consume less protein to lessen the load on your kidneys.

Fats: Transport vitamins K, E, D, and A to your cells. They produce the hormones testosterone and estrogen. Some fats contain fatty acids that are good for your skin.

There are two types of fats: unsaturated and saturated. Meat and dairy products are saturated fats. Too much of these fats can elevate your cholesterol; this cholesterol is what causes heart disease and clogged arteries. The food and drug administration recommends reducing your saturated fat intake. Nuts, fish, and certain oils are good sources of unsaturated fats and all help to reduce cholesterol. Trans fats will raise cholesterol levels, just like saturated fats. The FDA recommends selecting foods that are low in saturated and trans fats.

Sodium, potassium, and phosphorus: These are the three main minerals balanced by the kidneys. As chronic kidney disease gets worse, some foods will need to be avoided as your kidneys are already unable to remove the excess from these minerals. Blood tests will be conducted to monitor the levels of these minerals.

Sodium: If you have high blood pressure and are experiencing the early stages of renal disease, you need a low sodium diet. Your kidneys cannot get rid of excess fluid and sodium from your body whilst experiencing kidney disease. To help identify salt in foods, look for ingredients on the label such as baking powder, sodium, or brine. Generally, children and adults should eat less than 2,300 mg of sodium a day.

- **Kidney disease stage 1 and 2** = 1–3.5g per day
- **Kidney disease stage 3 - 4** = 1–2.5g per day
- **Kidney disease stage 5** = 1–2g per day

Potassium: To keep potassium levels in your blood at normal levels, kidneys generally eliminate excess potassium in your urine. When experiencing kidney disease, they can no longer do this effectively.

Hyperkalemia (or high potassium levels) occurs in the later stages of kidney disease. Symptoms of high potassium are a slow pulse, numbness, weakness, and nausea.

- **Kidney disease stage 1 and 2** = 2–5g per day
- **Kidney disease stage 3 - 4** =2–4g per day
- **Kidney disease stage 5** = 2–2.5 per day

Phosphorus: Since your kidneys can no longer remove phosphorus from your blood and urine, hyperphosphatemia or high phosphorus may become a problem during stage 4 or 5 kidney disease.

- **Kidney disease stage 1 and 2** = up to 1000mg per day
- **Kidney disease stage 3–4** (GFR of 25–90+) = p to 1000mg per day
- **Kidney disease stage 4** (GFR of 15–25) = up to 750mg per day
- **Kidney disease stage 4** (GFR of 5–15) = up to 7mg per kg of body weight

HOW TO REDUCE YOUR PHOSPHORUS INTAKE?

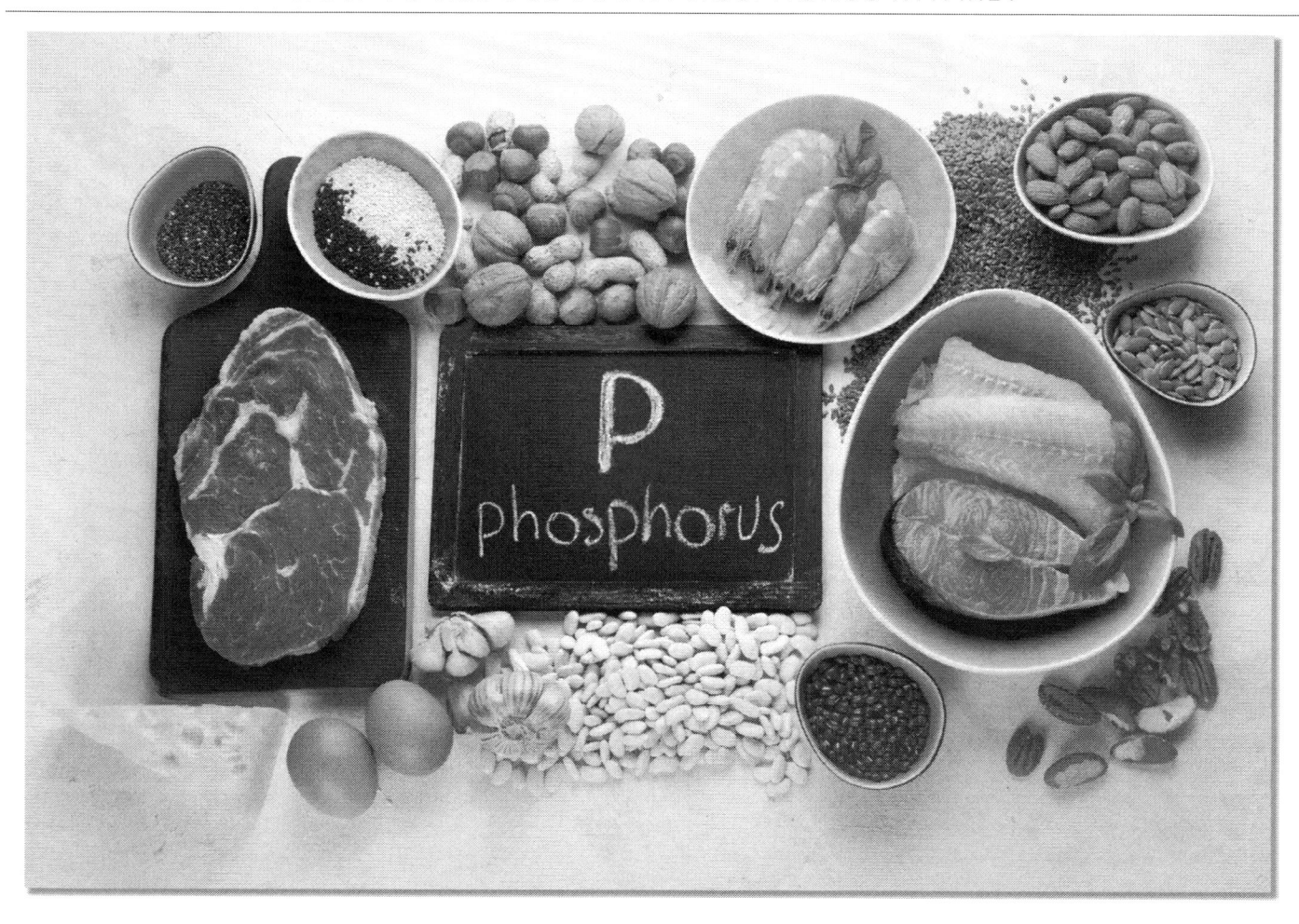

The entire philosophy of lowering phosphorus levels that should be regulated by your kidneys is to lower the intake of foods that are rich in this mineral. We don't recommend completely letting go of phosphorus-rich food groups as your body still needs phosphorus regardless of the state of your kidneys. Consult with your doctor to find out more about phosphorus levels in your blood so you would know which food you may need to give up on.

Foods that normally have high concentrations of phosphorus are meat, cheese, dairy, seeds, soda, seeds, and fast foods, so you may want to watch out for these food groups and make sure that your overall consumption of protein and dairy is restricted and limited just as it is the case with foods rich in sodium and potassium.

In case phosphorus levels found in your blood are higher than recommended according to your physician you are more likely to be advised to cut on meat and dairy portions, while meat also contains high concentrations of potassium.

The best way of monitoring quantities of phosphorus, potassium, and sodium you are ingesting through your everyday diet is to limit the food groups that contain high concentrations of these minerals.

Besides limiting foods that contain high levels of these minerals, you can also limit phosphorus introduced to your organism by cutting on portions that contain food that is high in phosphorus, sodium, or potassium.

Make sure to get familiar with which food groups contain the highest concentrations of phosphorus, while eating fresh veggies and fruit may help you in case you have increased phosphorus in your blood. Food that has more than 120 mg of phosphorus per serving is considered to be high-phosphorus food and should be introduced to your diet in limited amounts and in smaller portions, as well as it is the case with foods that are rich in potassium and sodium

Phosphorus represents an essential mineral that serves the purpose of maintaining bone structure and taking care of bone cell development. Phosphorus has more roles in our organism as an essential mineral, working on connective tissue and enabling muscle movement.

However, when concentrations of this mineral in your organism are too high as kidneys are unable to level phosphorus levels due to slow and damaged renal functions, redundant phosphorus becomes dangerous and may cause further health complications and aid in the progression of your chronic kidney's disease. Once phosphorus levels in your blood have surpassed recommended concentrations, the otherwise useful mineral becomes dangerous for your health as phosphorus then draws calcium from your bones, making the bones weak.

Common signs that appear as symptoms at kidney patients who have increased levels of phosphorus in their blood can appear in the form of heart calcification, weak and easily breakable bones, muscle pain, as well as calcification of skin and joints, as well as blood vessel calcification. With high levels of phosphorus that damaged kidneys are not able to eject from your blood, calcium builds up and can affect your lungs, eyes, heart, and blood vessels, altogether bringing more damage to your renal functions that are already weakened.

That is why watching out for phosphorus levels besides monitoring levels of potassium and sodium is essential for your renal health and can be easily conducted through a suitable diet such as a renal diet that originally prescribes low-sodium and low-potassium intake on a daily basis.

Just as it is the case with potassium and sodium, phosphorus is a mineral found in many different food groups, which means that the intake of this essential mineral can be monitored through food consumption.

HOW TO MONITOR YOUR POTASSIUM LEVELS?

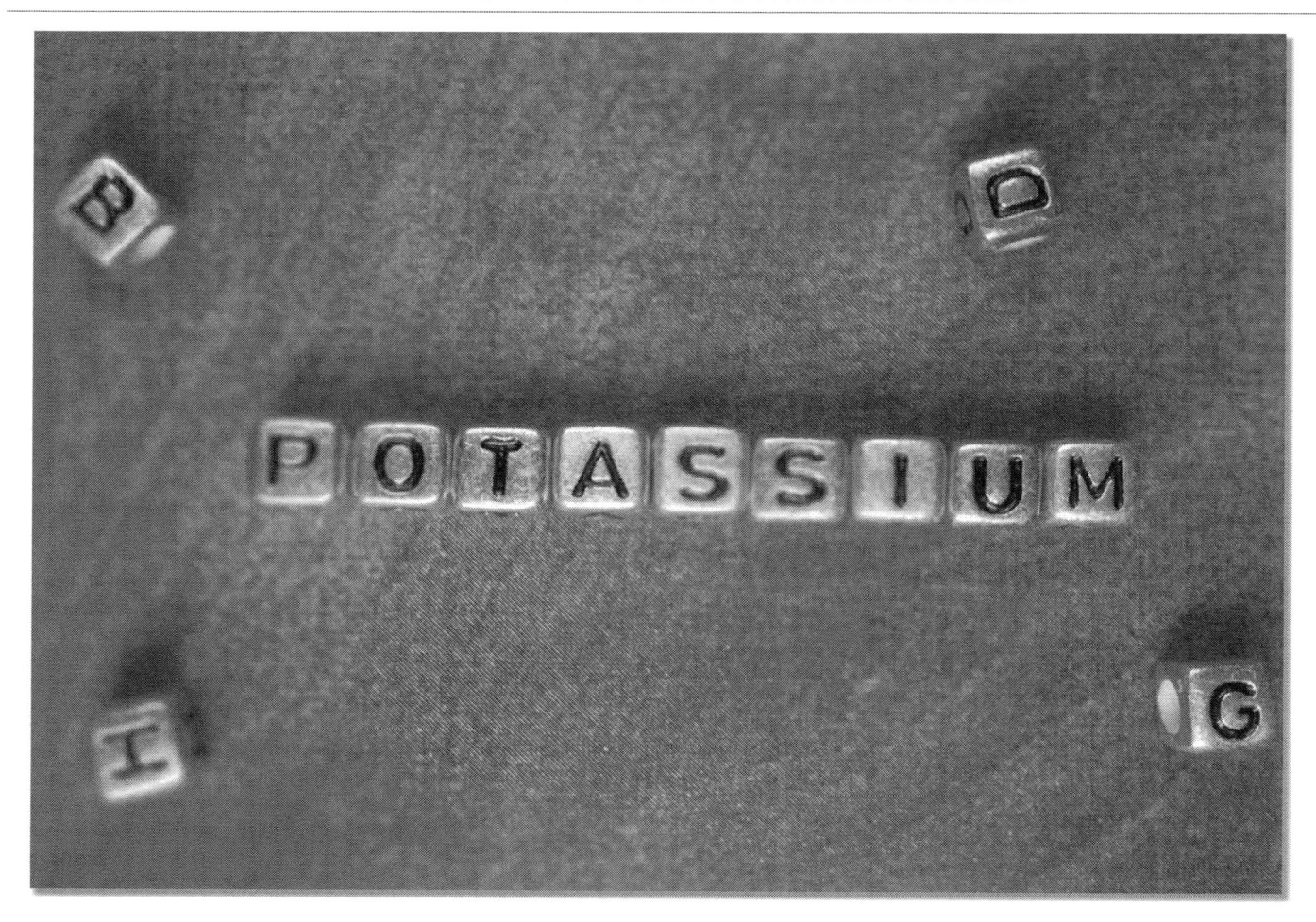

Potassium is a mineral and electrolyte that regulates metabolism and fluid levels and helps your muscles, kidneys, and heart function properly, but only in the right doses—it depends on how well your kidneys are working and whether you are taking medications that affect potassium levels.

In the early stages of kidney disease, potassium levels are usually normal.

If your potassium level is above normal during stages 1, 2, or 3 of CKD, your physician will probably conduct a blood test to help determine the cause and whether you need to make any dietary changes. If you are receiving dialysis, your potassium intake should be limited to 2,000 to 3,000 milligrams per day (see Calculate Your Intake). Excess potassium can harm the heart muscle and cause an irregular heartbeat or difficulty breathing, so maintaining the right balance is essential.

Potassium in Common Foods

LOW POTASSIUM (Less than 150 mg/serving)	MEDIUM POTASSIUM (151–250 mg/serving)	HIGH POTASSIUM (More than 251 mg/serving)
Alfalfa seeds, sprouted, raw	Apple, without skin, 1 large	Apricot, 1 cup
Apple juice	Apricot, halves, 1 medium	Artichoke, 1 medium
Applesauce, sweetened	Apricots, in heavy syrup, drained	Avocado
Bagel, 1 plain (4-inch diameter)	Asparagus, boiled, 5 spears	Bamboo shoots, cooked
Beans, green, frozen	Beans, green, boiled, 1 cup	Banana, 1 small
Blueberries	Blackberries, 1 cup	Beans, black, mature, boiled
Cabbage, shredded, boiled	Broccoli, frozen, 1 cup	Beans, dried
Carrot, baby raw, 1 medium	Brussels sprouts, boiled	Beans, Lima, large, mature, boiled, 1/3 cup
Cherries, sour canned, in syrup	Carrots, sliced, 1 cup	Beans, pinto, mature, boiled
Coffee, 1 cup	Cereal, All-Bran	Beans, refried, canned
Cranberries, dried	Cherries, 10 sweet	Beets, cooked
Cranberry juice	Chickpeas, dried, boiled	Cabbage, Chinese, cooked
Cranberry sauce, canned	Collards, chopped, frozen	Cantaloupe, cubed, 1 cup
Eggplant, boiled	Corn, yellow, boiled, 1 ear	Chard, Swiss, boiled, 1/3 cup
Fig, raw, 1 medium	Date, dried, 1 date	Chocolate
Ginger ale, 12 ounces	Elderberries	Dates, Medjool
Grapes	Grapefruit, ½ medium	Fruits, dried
Lemon, 1 medium	Grapefruit juice	Mango, pieces, 1 cup
Lime, 1 medium	Grape juice, 1 cup	Milk, 1%, 1 cup
Mustard greens, frozen	Honeydew melon, pieces	Milk, soy, 1 cup

Oatmeal, regular	Kiwifruit, 1 medium	Milk, whole, 1 cup
Okra, cooked	Leeks, 1 raw	Molasses, 1 tablespoon
Onions, raw, diced	Mustard greens, cooked, ¾ cup	Mushrooms, cooked, 1 cup
Parsley, raw, 10 sprigs	Onion, chopped, boiled	Nectarine, 1 medium
Peaches, canned, in syrup, drained	Orange, 1 medium	Nuts, mixed, 2 ounces
Pears, canned, in syrup, drained	Peach, 1 small	Orange juice, fresh
Peppers, sweet, cooked	Pear, 1 medium	Papaya, 1 small
Pineapple, pieces	Peppers, hot chile	Plantain, sliced, cooked
Plum, 1 medium	Peppers, sweet, raw	Pomegranate, 1 small
Popcorn, buttered	Pineapple, canned	Pomegranate juice
Prunes, dried, 1 prune	Pineapple juice	Potatoes, white, baked, 1 medium
Radicchio, raw, shredded	Prickly pear, 1 medium	Raisins, seedless, 1.5-ounce box
Raspberries	Prunes, canned, 5 prunes	Sapodilla, 1 medium
Rhubarb, cooked with sugar	Radishes, raw, sliced, 1 cup	Sauerkraut, undrained, 1 cup
Rice, white, enriched, 1 cup cooked	Raspberries, frozen, sweetened, 1 cup	Spinach, cooked
Spaghetti, enriched, cooked	Scallions, chopped, raw, 1 cup	Succotash, boiled
Spinach, raw, chopped	Squash, summer	Sweet potatoes, boiled
Tea, black, 8 ounces	Strawberries, whole, 1 cup	Tomato, 1 medium
Turnips, white, cubed	Tangerine, 1 large	Tomato paste, canned, ¼ cup
Water chestnuts, canned	Tortillas, corn, 4 (6-inch diameter)	Tomato sauce, canned, ¼ cup
Watermelon, pieces	Turnip greens, chopped	Water chestnuts, raw

*One serving = ½ cup unless otherwise noted.

HOW TO DECREASE YOUR SODIUM INTAKE?

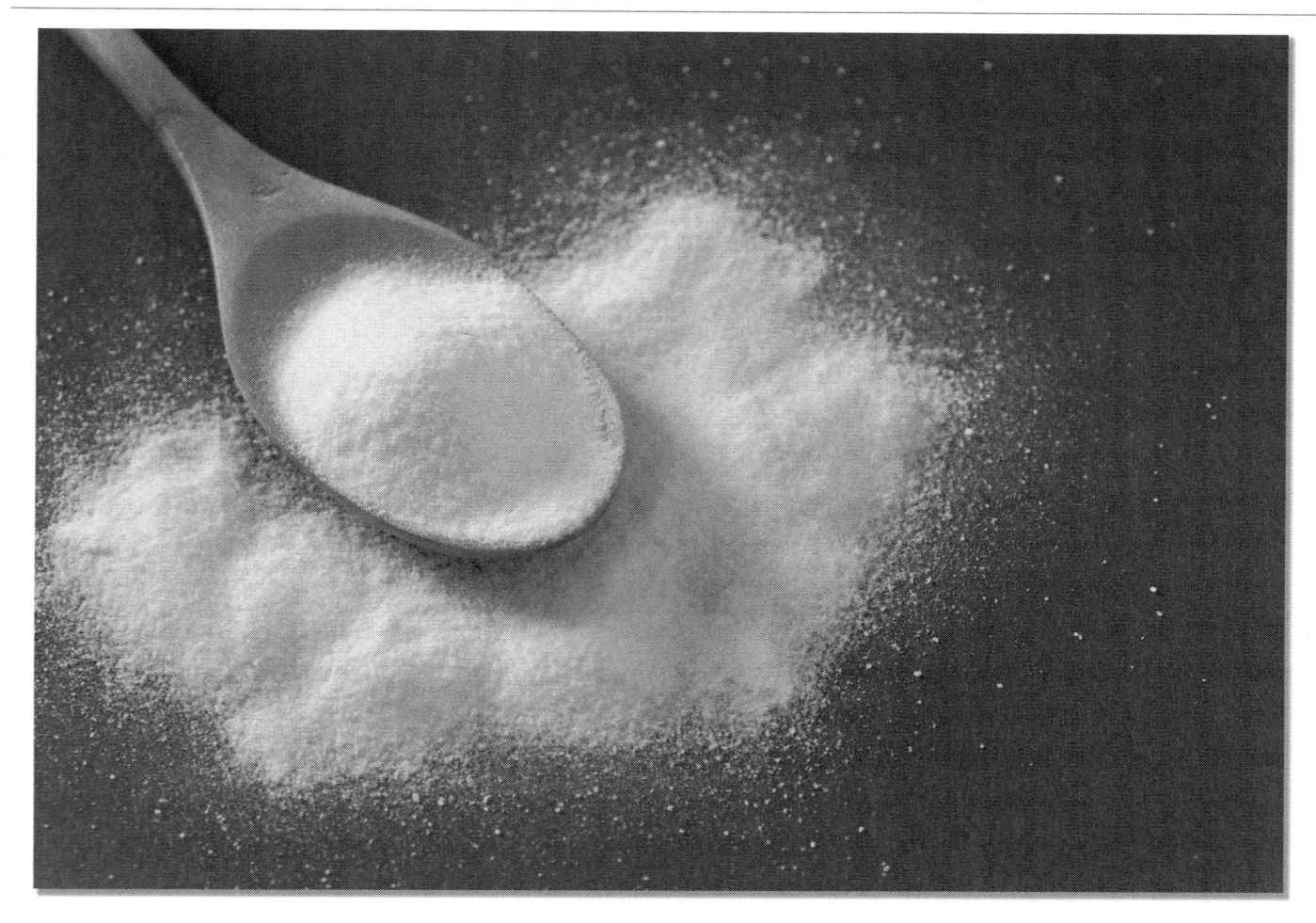

Sodium is a type of minerals that are found in most natural foods. While most people think of salt and sodium interchangeably, however, salt is a compound of sodium and chloride. The food we eat may contain salt or other forms of sodium, it is still the most commonly used type of seasoning, and it takes time to get used to reducing salt in your diet. Though, a higher amount of sodium can be found in processed foods which are due to the added salt in it.

Sodium is among the body's three major electrolytes (the other two are chloride and potassium). The work of the electrolyte is to control the fluids going in and out of the body's cells and tissues. So, the following are the contributions of sodium to the body:

- **Regulating** muscle contraction and nerve function
- **Balancing** how much fluid the body eliminates or keep
- **Regulating** the acid-base balance of the blood
- **Regulating** blood volume and blood pressure

REASONS WHY YOU SHOULD MONITOR YOUR SODIUM INTAKE

Taking too much sodium can be harmful to people suffering from kidney disease, this is because their kidneys cannot properly eliminate excess sodium and fluid from their body. Because as sodium and fluids build up in the tissues and bloodstreams, they can cause the following to happen:

- Edema: swelling in the hands, legs, and face.
- High blood pressure
- Increased thirst
- Inadequate breathing: fluids can build up in the lungs and makes it hard to breathe.
- Heart failure: the excess fluid in the bloodstream can make the heart over-work, and become enlarged and weak

HOW TO MONITOR YOUR SODIUM INTAKE?

- Always pay attention to serving sizes
- Avoid processed foods
- Compare different brands and use items that are lowest in sodium
- Cook at home and avoid adding salt to foods
- Use fresh meat instead of packaged meats
- Avoid foods that contain more than 300mg sodium per serving (or 600mg for a frozen dinner)
- Limit your sodium consumption per meal to 300mg, and in the case of snacks, limit it to 150mg
- Do not put salt on food when you eat
- Choose spices that do not list salt in their description (you can select garlic powder rather than garlic salt, onion salt)
- Choose fresh fruits and vegetables or canned and frozen produce that doesn't contain salt. These are usually chicken breasts, steaks, pork chops, pork tenderloin, or burgers.
- Always read food labels and check if sodium is listed in the content.

If you are in the early stages of chronic kidney failure (i.e., stages 1 - 4), you will need to make some dietary changes if you have high blood pressure or if you are holding fluids.

If you have stage 5 chronic kidney disease and need dialysis, you will need to follow a low sodium diet and not consume more than 1,500 milligrams of sodium per day, which is equivalent to about one tablespoon of salt. (It is important to note that one tablespoon of salt per day is the total amount of sodium that is allowed to you, which includes all foods, plus added salt.)

FOOD THAT YOU MUST AVOID

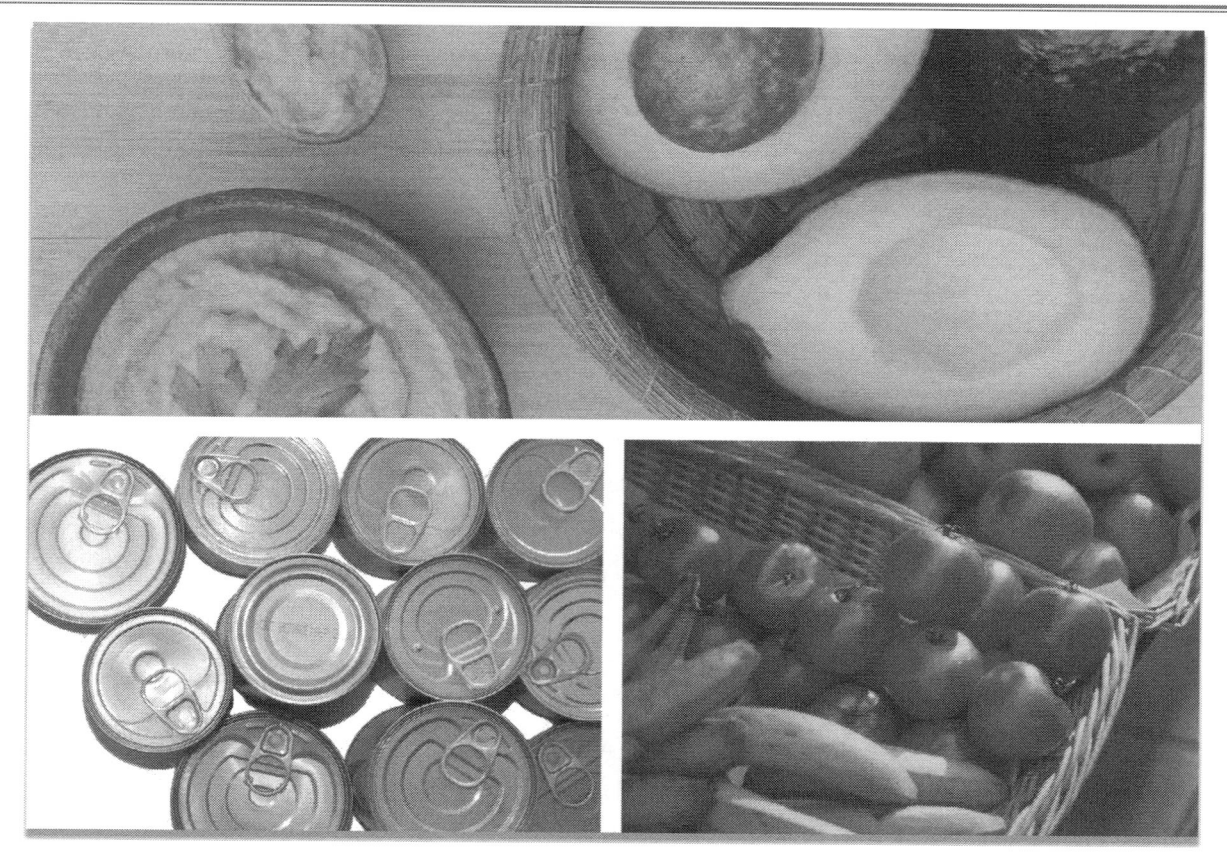

In order to follow the renal diet that will support kidney function and not disrupt it, you may want to avoid consuming the following foods:

- Avocado – while they are healthy, avocadoes are abundant in potassium
- Canned foods – contain high amounts of sodium
- Whole-wheat bread – due to its phosphorus and potassium content
- Brown rice – high in potassium and phosphorus
- Bananas – abundant in potassium
- Dairy – a natural source of phosphorus, potassium, protein
- Oranges (and OJ) – a rich source of potassium
- Processed meat – contain high amounts of salt
- Olives, pickles, and relish – too much salt
- Apricots – high in potassium
- Potatoes and sweet potatoes – contain high levels of potassium
- Tomatoes – high in potassium
- Instant, packaged, and premade meals – abundant in sodium
- Spinach, beet greens, Swiss chard – contain high amounts of potassium
- Prunes, raisins, and dates – abundant in potassium
- Crackers, chips, pretzels, and other snacks – high in salt

NOTE: some foods such as potatoes and sweet potatoes can be leached or soaked to reduce potassium content.

FOODS TO EAT

When it comes to renal diet, you need to opt for foods that are low in sodium, potassium, phosphorus, and protein. Below, you can see the list of foods that are considered the most beneficial for people with kidney disease:

- Cauliflower – anti-inflammatory properties, abundant in vitamin C, vitamin K, and folate
- Blueberries – nutrient-rich and abundant in antioxidants that decrease the risk of diabetes, heart disease, and cognitive decline
- Sea bass – high-quality protein and a good source of Omega-3 fatty acids
- Red grapes – rich in vitamin C and other valuable nutrients
- Egg whites – a kidney-friendly source of protein
- Garlic – a delicious alternative to salt
- Buckwheat – nutritious, rich in fiber, magnesium, iron, and B vitamins
- Olive oil – phosphorus-free
- Bulgur – kidney-friendly alternative to whole grains
- Cabbage – a great source of vitamin K, vitamin C, and B-complex vitamins
- Skinless chicken – contains less phosphorus, sodium, and potassium than chicken with skin on (remember, an adequate amount of protein is important for your health)
- Bell peppers – low in potassium
- Onions – sodium-free flavor for renal diet
- Arugula – nutrient-dense green vegetable low in potassium
- Macadamia nuts – low in phosphorus
- Radish – low in potassium and phosphorus
- Turnip – excellent replacement for high-potassium vegetables such as potatoes
- Pineapple – low potassium content
- Cranberries – contain nutrients that prevent bacteria from sticking to the lining of the bladder and urinary tract to cut the risk of infections
- Shiitake mushrooms – a plant-based meat substitute
- Apples – high in fiber and anti-inflammatory compounds

FLUIDS AND JUICES FOR HEALTHY KIDNEYS

Management of kidney disease also requires paying attention to fluid intake and the things you drink. For example, you should definitely avoid soda, especially dark-colored cola. But here are some drinks you should include in your lifestyle:

- Cranberry juice – beneficial for urinary and kidney health
- Lemon- and lime-based or other citrus juice – kidney stone prevention
- Water – allows kidneys to filter waste and toxins from the blood
- Stinging nettle tea – antioxidant-rich, reduces inflammation

Now that you know what to eat and avoid on the renal diet, it's time to start cooking.

SHOPPING LIST, AND MEAL PLAN

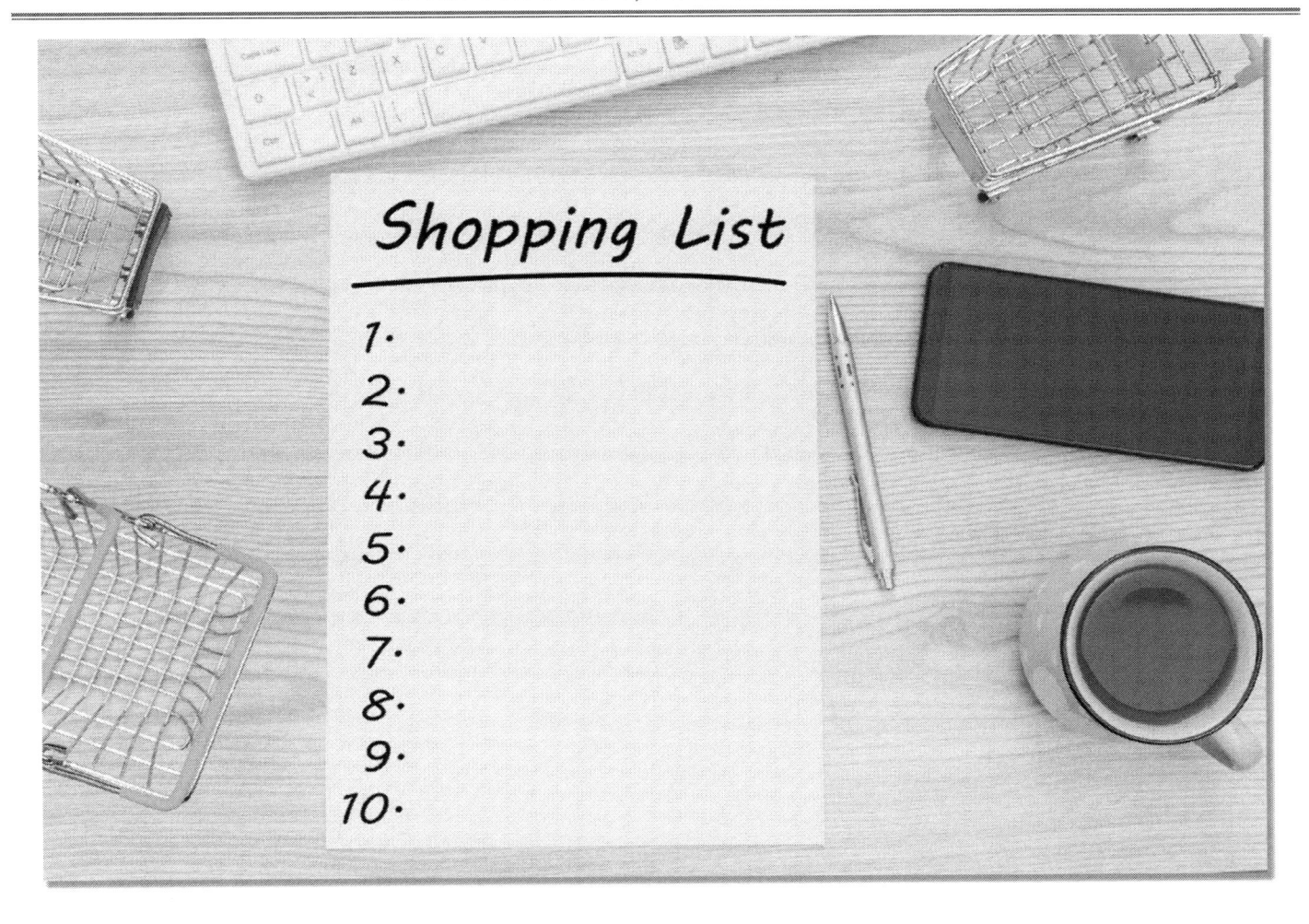

RENAL DIET SHOPPING LIST

Vegetables:

- Arugula (raw)
- Alfalfa sprouts
- Bamboo shoots
- Asparagus
- Beans - pinto, wax, fava, green
- Bean sprouts
- Bitter melon (balsam pear)
- Beet greens (raw)
- Broccoli
- Broad beans (boiled, fresh)
- Cactus
- Cabbage - red, swamp, Napa/ Suey Choy, skunk
- Carrots
- Calabash
- Celery
- Cauliflower
- Chayote
- Celeriac (cooked)
- Collard greens
- Chicory
- Cucumber
- Corn
- Okra
- Onions
- Pepitas
- (Green) Peas
- Peppers
- Radish
- Radicchio
- Seaweed
- Rapini (raw)
- Shallots
- Spinach (raw)
- Snow peas
- Dandelion greens (raw)
- Daikon
- Plant Leaves
- Drumstick
- Endive
- Eggplant
- Fennel bulb
- Escarole
- Fiddlehead greens
- Ferns

- Hearts of Palm
- GaiLan
- Irishmoss
- Hominy
- Jicama, raw
- Jew's Ear
- Leeks
- Kale(raw)
- Mushrooms (raw white)
- Lettuce(raw)
- Nopales
- Mustard greens
- Swiss chard (raw)
- Squash
- Turnip
- Tomatillos (raw)
- Watercress
- Turnip greens
- Wax beans
- Water chestnuts (canned)
- Winter melon
- Wax gourd
- Zucchini (raw)

Fruits:
- Acerola Cherries
- Apple
- Blackberries
- Asian Pear
- Boysenberries
- Blueberries
- Cherries
- Casaba melon
- Clementine
- Chokeberries
- Crabapples
- Cloudberries
- Feijoa
- Cranberries (fresh)
- Grapefruit
- Gooseberries
- Pomegranate
- Grapes
- Rambutan
- Quince
- Rhubarb
- Raspberries (fresh or frozen)

- Jujubes
- Golden Berry
- Kumquat
- Jackfruit
- Lingonberries
- Lemon
- Loganberries
- Lime
- Lychees
- Longans
- Mango
- Mandarin orange
- Peach
- Mangosteen
- Pineapple
- Pear
- Plum
- Pitanga
- Strawberries
- Rose-apple
- Tangerine
- Tangelo
- Watermelon

Bread products:

Packaged bread:

- Dimpflmeier Holzofen Art Brot-Real Stone Bread
- Country Harvest Vitality White with Whole Wheat
- Stonemill Sourdough Classic French
- Dimpflmeier Viking French Stick Bread
- Wonder White Thin Sandwich
- Wonder White + Fibre Bread
- Naan Bread
- Chapati/Roti
- Pita Bread
- Dempster's Smart White with 16 Whole Grains
- Wonder White with Fibre English Muffin
- Silver Hills Bakery Little Big, Steady Eddie

Packaged Bagels:

- Dempster's Original Bagels
- Stonemill Swiss Muesli Bagels

Hamburger/Hot Dog Buns:

- Wonder White Hamburger Bun
- Wonder White Hot Dog buns
- Dempster's Hot Dog Bun

Tortillas and Taco Shells:

- Old El Paso Flour Tortillas
- White flour or corn-based tortillas
- Old El Paso Taco Shells

Fresh Meat, Seafood, and Poultry:

- Chicken
- Beef and Ground Beef
- Goat
- Duck
- Wild Game
- Pork
- Lamb
- Veal
- Turkey
- Fish

Milk, Eggs, and Dairy:

Milk:

- Milk (½-1 cup/day)

Non-Dairy Milk:

- Almond Fresh (Original, Unsweetened, Vanilla)
- Almond Breeze (Original, Vanilla, Vanilla Unsweetened, Original Unsweetened)
- Silk True Almond Beverage (Unsweetened Original, Original, Vanilla, Unsweetened Vanilla)
- Good Karma Flax Delight (Vanilla, Original, Unsweetened)
- Rice Dream Rice Drink (Vanilla Classic, Non-Enriched Original Classic)
- Silk Soy Beverage (Original, Vanilla, Unsweetened)
- Natura Organic Fortified Rice Beverage (Original, Vanilla)
- PC Organics Fortified Rice Beverage

Coffee Creamer:

- Nestle Coffee-Mate (Original Fat-Free, Original, Original Low Fat)

Cheese:

- Feta
- Brie
- Goat Cheese, Soft
- Grated Parmesan Cheese
- Nanak Paneer President's Choice Bocconcini
- Liberte Fresh Cheese, Crème Fraiche
- Western Pressed Dry Cottage Cheese 0.1% or 0.5%, No Salt
- Trestelle Bocconcini, 40% Light Bocconcini, Mascarpone
- Lucerne Cottage Cheese, 2% No-Added-Salt

Other Dairy Products:

- Non-Hydrogenated Margarine (Salt-Free or Regular)
- Butter (Unsalted or Regular)
- Whipping Cream
- Sour Cream
- Whipped Cream

Eggs:

- Egg Beaters
- Fresh eggs, all types

Tofu:

- Tofu (soft)

Salt-Free Seasonings:

- McCormack Salt-Free Garlic and Herb, All-Purpose
- Clubhouse La Grille No Salt Added Chicken Seasoning, No Salt Added Steak Spice
- Allspice
- Anise
- Mrs. Dash
- Caraway seeds
- Celery seeds
- Cardamom
- Basil
- Bay Leaves
- Coriander
- Curry powder
- Cumin
- Chives
- Cinnamon
- Cloves
- Cilantro
- Garlic powder
- Ginger
- Dill
- Fennel
- Fenugreek
- Nutmeg
- Mace
- Mustard
- Marjoram
- Paprika
- Pepper (Black or Cayenne)
- Parsley
- Onion powder/flakes
- Oregano
- Rosemary
- Poultry seasoning
- Poppy seeds
- Tarragon
- Turmeric
- Thyme
- Saffron
- Savory
- Sage

MEAL PLAN

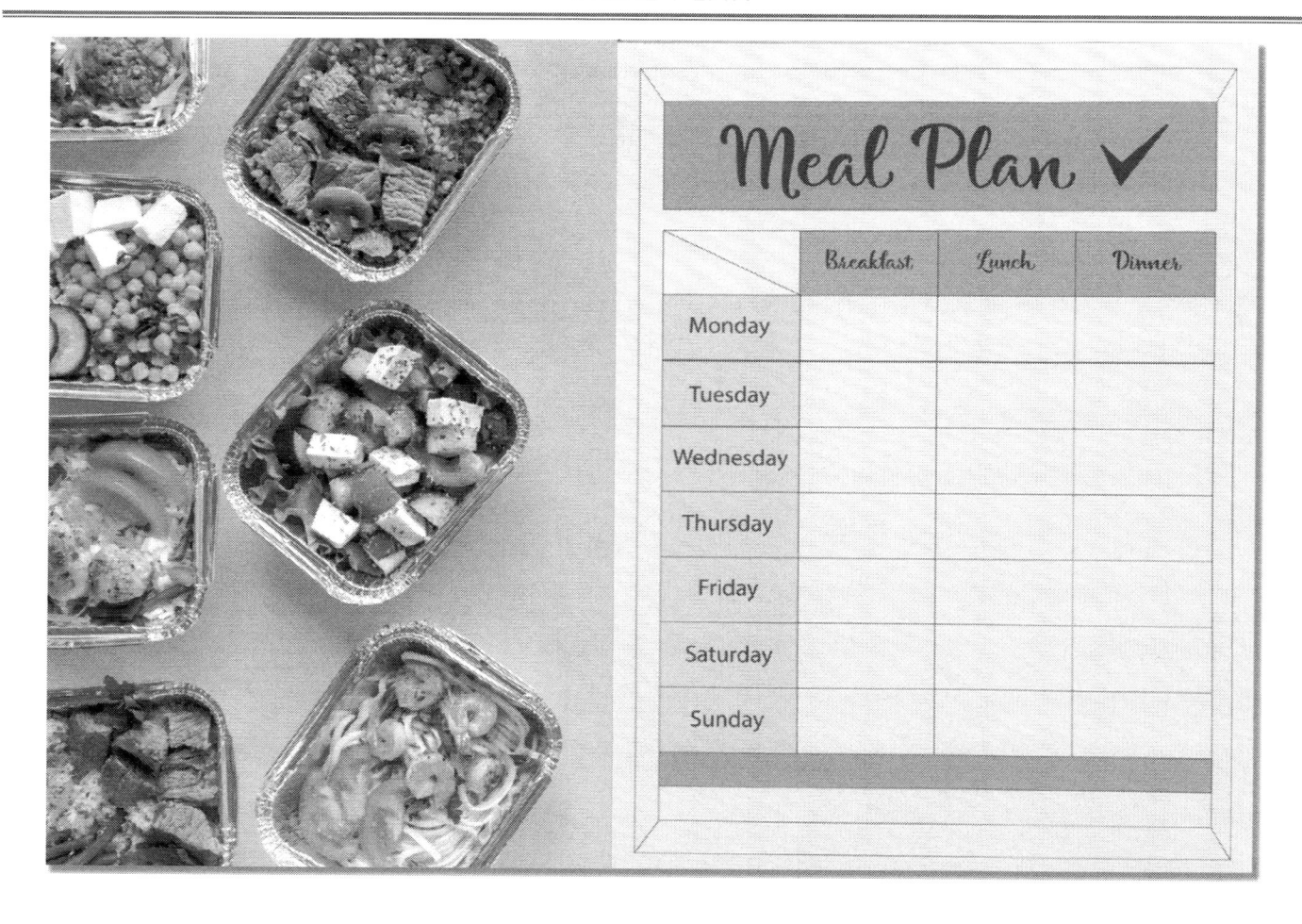

Meal Plan ✓

	Breakfast	Lunch	Dinner
Monday			
Tuesday			
Wednesday			
Thursday			
Friday			
Saturday			
Sunday			

WEEK 1 MEAL PLAN

	Breakfast	**Lunch**	**Dinner**
Monday	Green Breakfast Soup	Salad with Vinaigrette	Lemon Sprouts
Tuesday	Peach Berry Parfait	Salad with Lemon Dressing	Lemon and Broccoli Platter
Wednesday	Open-Faced Bagel Breakfast Sandwich	Shrimp with Salsa	Chicken Liver Stew
Thursday	Bulgur Bowl with Strawberries and Walnuts	Cauliflower Soup	Mushroom Cream Soup
Friday	Overnight Oats Three Ways	Cabbage Stew	Garlic Soup
Saturday	Buckwheat Pancakes	Baked Haddock	Simple Lamb Chops
Sunday	Peach Berry Parfait	Herbed Chicken	Garlic and Butter- Flavored Cod

WEEK 2 MEAL PLAN

	Breakfast	**Lunch**	**Dinner**
Monday	Broccoli Basil Quiche	Pesto Pork Chops	Parsley Scallops
Tuesday	Asparagus Frittata	Vegetable Curry	Blackened Chicken
Wednesday	Poached Eggs with Cilantro Butter	Grilled Steak with Salsa	Spicy Paprika Lamb Chops
Thursday	Tasty Pancakes	Eggplant and Red Pepper Soup	Cabbage and Beef Fry
Friday	Slow-Cooked Oats	Persian Chicken	Mushroom and Olive Sirloin Steak
Saturday	Brown Muffins	Pork Souvlaki	Kale and Garlic Platter
Sunday	Papaya Orange Smoothie	Chicken Stew	Blistered Beans and Almond

WEEK 3 MEAL PLAN

	Breakfast	Lunch	Dinner
Monday	Easy Corn Pudding	Baked Flounder	Tuna Casserole
Tuesday	Sliced Apple Cookies	Caraway Cabbage and Rice	Oregano Salmon with Crunchy Crust
Wednesday	Chocolate Spring Muffins	Orzo and Vegetables	Sardine Fish Cakes
Thursday	Savory Spring Muffins	Chicken and Asparagus Pasta	Cajun Catfish
Friday	Pita with Egg & Curry	Hawaiian Rice	Teriyaki Tuna
Saturday	Hot Vanilla Cereals	Shrimp Fried Rice	Chicken Noodle Soup
Sunday	Aromatic Carrot Cream	Vegetarian Egg Fried Rice	Beef Stew with Apple Cider
Monday	Mushrooms Velvet Soup	Autumn Orzo Salad	Chicken Chili

WEEK 4 MEAL PLAN

	Breakfast	Lunch	Dinner
Monday	Easy Lettuce Wraps	Blackened Shrimp and Pineapple Salad	Tofu Stir Fry
Tuesday	Spaghetti with Pesto	Green Pepper Slaw	Broccoli Pancake
Wednesday	Spiced Wraps	Cranberries and Couscous Salad	Tangy Whole Roasted Sea Bass with Oregano
Thursday	Poached Asparagus and Egg	Tuna Salad	Pan-Seared Salmon with Lemon Dressing
Friday	Apple Turnover	Roasted Vegetable Salad	Grilled Steak served with Creamy Peanut Sauce
Saturday	Egg Drop Soup	Chicken Pita Pizza	Lean Steak with Oregano-Lemon Chimichurri & Arugula Salad
Sunday	Roasted Pepper Soup	Chicken Wraps	Herbed London Broil
Monday	Assorted Fresh Fruit Juice	Mexican Chicken Pizza	Ground Beef Tacos

DIETARY STAGES OF RENAL DIET

If you are diagnosed with chronic kidney disease, you will discover that unfortunately the condition gradually gets worse over time.

A renal diet is an eating plan tailored to the individual's needs and can vary depending on their stage of chronic kidney disease (CKD). Generally, it includes limiting sodium, phosphorus, and protein intake, as well as increasing the intake of healthy fats, fruits, and vegetables. It also includes drinking plenty of fluids and avoiding certain foods and beverages that can worsen kidney function. Following a renal diet can help reduce the symptoms and progression of CKD, as well as reduce the risk of developing further complications.

Chronic kidney disease (CKD) is a condition that affects the kidneys and is classified into five stages, ranging from mild (Stage 1) to severe (Stage 5).

The stages are determined by the estimated glomerular filtration rate (**eGFR**), which is a measure of the kidney's ability to filter waste and toxins from the blood.

A low eGFR means the kidneys are not functioning properly and CKD is present.

In **Stage 1**, the eGFR level is 90 or above, and there are usually no symptoms.

In **Stage 2**, the eGFR level is between 60 and 89, and there may be mild symptoms such as fatigue, nausea, and loss of appetite.

In **Stage 3**, the eGFR level is between 30 and 59, and there may be more severe symptoms such as swelling in the legs or feet, difficulty sleeping, and increased urination.

In **Stage 4**, the eGFR level is between 15 and 29, and the condition is considered to be severe.

Stage 5 is the most severe stage of the condition. At this stage, the eGFR level is below 15, and the condition has progressed to end-stage kidney disease (ESKD).

Symptoms of Stage 5 CKD can include swelling in the face, feet, and hands; severe fatigue; loss of appetite; difficulty sleeping; nausea; and vomiting. In this stage, dialysis or a kidney transplant is usually necessary to keep the patient healthy.

Managing Chronic Kidney Disease is important to ensure that the condition does not worsen.

STAGE ONE

This is the mildest stage of the condition. At this stage, the estimated glomerular filtration rate (GFR) is 90 or above and there are usually no symptoms.

The first stage of a renal diet is the most restrictive, as it aims to limit the intake of protein, potassium, and phosphorus. People in this stage may have a high creatinine level or have recently been diagnosed with kidney disease.

This stage is typically recommended for people with a creatinine level greater than 2.5 or for those who have recently been diagnosed with kidney disease. In this stage, protein intake is limited to 20-40 grams per day. High-potassium foods such as bananas, oranges, and potatoes are also restricted, as well as high-phosphorus foods like dairy products, nuts, and seeds.

STAGE TWO

Stage two kidney disease is a mild type of chronic kidney disease, with a glomerular filtration rate (GFR) is 60-89 mL/min.

The second stage is less restrictive than the first stage, and it aims to limit the intake of protein and potassium, but not phosphorus. People in this stage may have a moderately high creatinine level or be in the early stages of kidney disease.

This stage is typically recommended for people with a creatinine level between 1.5 and 2.5 or for those who are in the early stages of kidney disease. In this stage, protein intake is limited to 40-60 grams per day. High-potassium foods such as bananas, oranges, and potatoes are still restricted but high-phosphorus foods such as dairy products, nuts, and seeds are allowed in moderation.

STAGE THREE

The third stage is even less restrictive than the second stage, and it aims to limit the intake of protein only. People in this stage may have a relatively stable creatinine level or be in the later stages of kidney disease.

This stage is typically recommended for people with a creatinine level between 1 and 1.5 or for those who are in the later stages of kidney disease. In this stage, protein intake is limited to 60-80 grams per day. High-potassium and high-phosphorus foods are allowed in moderation.

STAGE FOUR

Stage four kidney disease is a severe type of chronic kidney disease, with a glomerular filtration rate: GFR = 15-29 mL/min.

The fourth stage is the least restrictive and aims to provide adequate nutrition for people with end-stage kidney disease who are on dialysis.

This stage is typically recommended for people on dialysis or with end-stage kidney disease. In this stage, protein intake is increased to 80-100 grams per day. High-potassium and high-phosphorus foods are allowed in moderation.

STAGE FIVE

Stage five kidney disease is an end-stage type of chronic kidney disease, with a glomerular filtration rate: GFR < 15 mL/min.

This stage is typically recommended for people who have had a kidney transplant. In this stage, protein intake is increased to 100-120 grams per day. High-potassium and high-phosphorus foods are allowed in moderation.

t's important to note that a renal diet should be individualized and closely monitored by a **renal dietitian**, and should be adjusted as the patient's kidney function changes over time. In addition, people with kidney disease may also have other health conditions, such as diabetes or heart disease, that will also need to be considered when developing their diet plan.

Additionally, it is important to limit the intake of salt, fluids (if patient has fluid overload), and alcohol, and to avoid processed foods, fried foods and foods that are high in saturated fat.

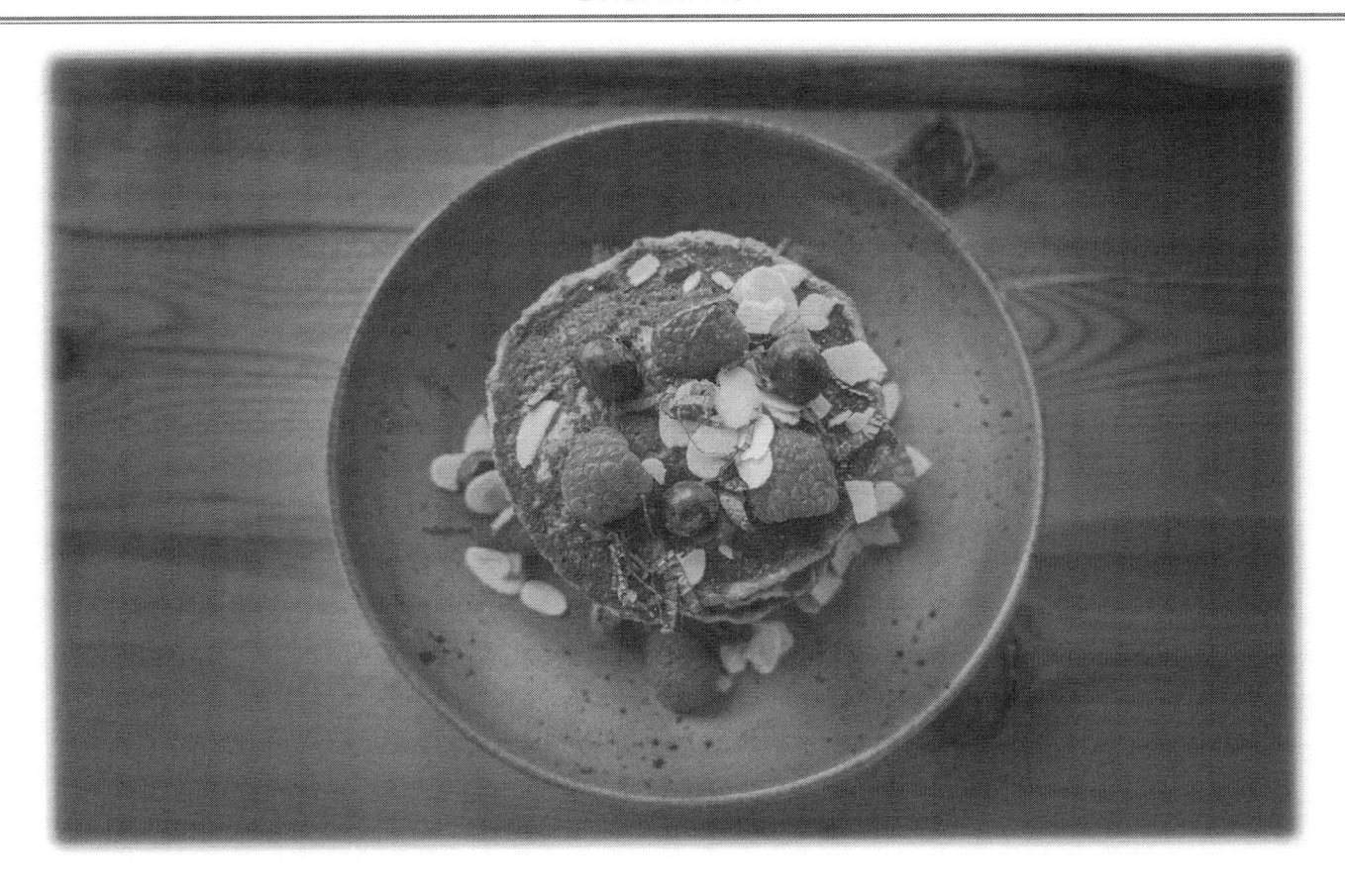

BREAKFAST

PEACH BERRY PARFAIT

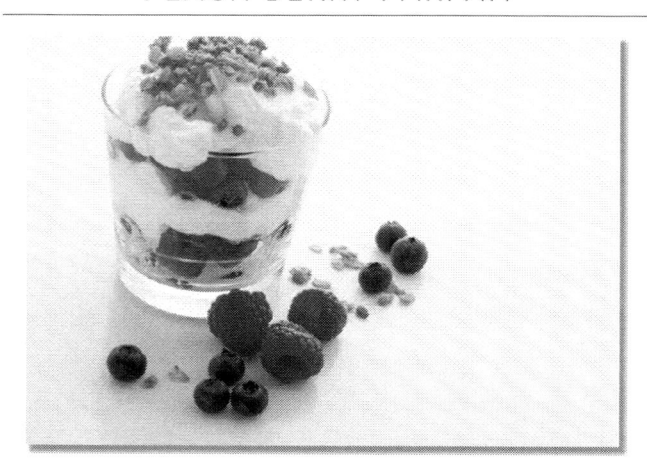

PREPARATION: 5 min.
COOKING TIME: -
SERVING: 2 People

Ingredients:

- 1 cup plain, non-sugar yogurt, split
- 1 teaspoon vanilla extract
- 1 small peach, diced
- ½ cup blueberries
- 2 ½ tablespoons walnut pieces

Directions:

1. In a small bowl, mix together the yogurt and vanilla.

2. Add 2 tablespoons of yogurt to each of 2 cups.

3. Divide the diced peach and the blueberries between the cups, and top with the remaining yogurt.

4. Sprinkle each cup with 1 tablespoon of walnut pieces.

Nutrition: Calories:191, Potassium: 327mg, Phosphorous:189mg, Protein:11g, Sodium:52mg, Fat:10g

OPEN-FACED BAGEL BREAKFAST SANDWICH

PREPARATION: 5 min.
COOKING TIME: 5 min.
SERVING: 2 People

Ingredients:

- 1 multigrain bagel, halved
- 2 tablespoons cream cheese, divided
- 2 slices tomato
- 1 slice red onion
- Freshly ground black pepper
- 1 cup microgreens

Directions:

1. In a toaster or oven, lightly toast the bagel.
2. Put a tablespoon of cream cheese on each half of the bagel,
3. Add 1 ½ tomato slice and a few onion rings to each half.
4. Season with the black pepper.
5. Top each half with ½ cup of microgreens and serve.

Nutrition: Calories:157, Potassium:164mg, Phosphorous:99mg, Protein:6g, Sodium:194 mg, Fat:6g

BULGUR BOWL WITH STRAWBERRIES AND WALNUTS

PREPARATION: 10 min.
COOKING TIME: 13 min.
SERVING: 4/5 People

Ingredients:

- 1 cup bulgur
- 1 cup strawberries, sliced
- 5 tablespoons (¼ cup) Homemade Rice Milk or unsweetened store-bought rice milk
- 3 teaspoons brown sugar
- 3 teaspoons extra-virgin olive oil
- 4/5 tablespoons (¼ cup) walnut pieces
- 5 tablespoons (¼ cup) cacao nibs (optional)

Directions:

1. In a small pot, combine the bulgur with 2 cups of water.
2. Bring to a simmer, reduce the heat and let simmer, covered, for 12 to 15 minutes, until tender.
3. Take it off the heat and drain any additional water.
4. In each of four bowls, add a quarter of the bulgur and top with ¼ cup of strawberries, 1 tablespoon of rice milk, 1 teaspoon of brown sugar, 1 teaspoon of olive oil, 1 tablespoon of walnut pieces, and 1 tablespoon of cacao nibs (if using).

Nutrition: Calories:190, Potassium:153 mg, Phosphorous: 66mg, Protein:4g, Sodium:13 mg, Fat:9g

OVERNIGHT OATS THREE WAYS

PREPARATION: 5 min.
COOKING TIME: 5 hours
SERVING: 2 People

Ingredients:

- ¾ cup Homemade Rice Milk or unsweetened store-bought rice milk
- ½ cup plain, unsweetened yogurt
- ½ cup rolled oats
- 1 tablespoon ground flaxseed
- 1 teaspoon vanilla extract
- 2 teaspoons honey

Directions:

1. In a medium bowl, mix the rice milk, yogurt, oats, flaxseed, vanilla, and honey.
2. Add the ingredients to make your preferred variation and stir to blend.
3. Divide between two jars.
4. Cover, and refrigerate for at least 4-5 hours or overnight.

Nutrition: Calories:196, Potassium:114 mg, Phosphorous: 99mg, Protein:8g, Sodium:63 mg, Fat:7g

BUCKWHEAT PANCAKES

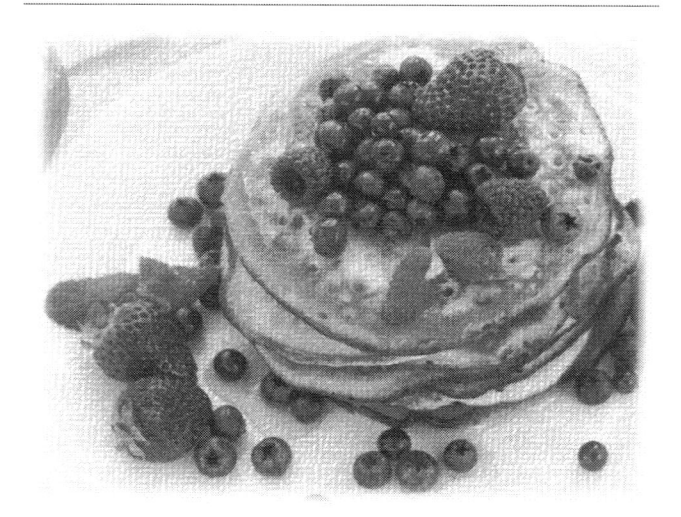

PREPARATION: 10 min.
COOKING TIME: 15 min.
SERVING: 4 People

Ingredients:

- 1¾ cups Homemade Rice Milk or unsweetened store-bought rice milk
- 2 ½ teaspoons white vinegar
- 1 ½ cup buckwheat flour
- Half a cup all-purpose flour
- 1 tablespoon sugar
- 2 tablespoons baking powder without phosphorus
- 1 large egg
- 1 ½ teaspoon vanilla extract
- For the skillet, use 2 tablespoons of butter.

Directions:

1. Combine the rice milk and vinegar in a small bowl. Let sit for 5 minutes.
2. In the meantime, combine the all-purpose flour and buckwheat flour in a large bowl.
3. Add the sugar and baking powder,
4. Stir to blend.
5. Add the egg and vanilla to the rice milk and stir to blend.
6. Add the wet ingredients to the dry and stir until just mixed.
7. In a large skillet over medium heat, melt 1½ teaspoons of butter. Use a ¼-cup measuring cup to scoop the batter into the skillet.
8. Cook for 2 to 4 minutes, until small bubbles form on the surface of the pancakes.
9. Flip and cook on the opposite side for 1 to 3 minutes
10. Place the pancakes on a dish for serving.

Nutrition: Calories:264, Potassium:399 mg, Phosphorous: 147mg, Protein:7g, Sodium:232 mg, Fat:9g

APPLE AND CINNAMON FRENCH TOAST STRATA

PREPARATION: 2 Hrs. 20 min.
COOKING TIME: 50 min.
SERVING: 12 People

Ingredients:

- 1 ½ medium apples peeled, cored, diced
- 1-pound cinnamon and raisin loaf, diced
- One teaspoon ground cinnamon
- ¼ cup pancake syrup
- Six tablespoons of melted unsalted butter
- One ¼ cup half-and-half creamer
- 8-9 ounces cream cheese, softened and cubed
- Eight large eggs
- One ¼ cup almond milk, unsweetened

Directions:

1. Take a 9x13 inches baking pan, grease it with oil, then layer half of the bread cubes on the bottom and scatter cream cheese evenly on the top.
2. Top cream cheese with the apple, sprinkle with cinnamon and then cover with the remaining bread cubes.
3. Crack eggs in a large bowl, add pancake syrup, butter, milk, and creamer, whisk until combined, pour this mixture evenly in the prepared casserole, cover it with plastic wrap, and then keep the casserole dish in the refrigerator for 2 hours.
4. When ready to cook, turn on the oven, set it to 325ºF, and preheat.
5. Then uncover casserole, bake for 45-50 minutes and when done, let it cool for 10 minutes and cut it into twelve 3x3 inches squares.
6. Add extra pancake syrup before serving.

Nutrition: Calories: 325, Fat: 20 g, Protein: 8 g, Carbohydrates: 28 g, Fiber: 1.9 g

BROCCOLI BASIL QUICHE

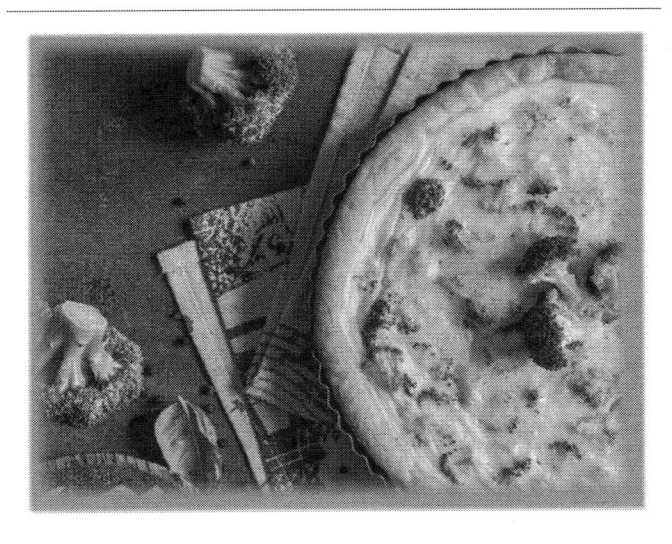

PREPARATION: 10 min.
COOKING TIME: 55 min.
SERVING: 8 People

Ingredients:

- 1 store-bought frozen piecrust
- 2 cups finely chopped broccoli
- 1 tomato, chopped
- 2 scallions, chopped
- 3 eggs, beaten
- 2 tablespoons chopped basil
- 1 cup Homemade Rice Milk or unsweetened store-bought rice milk
- ½ cup crumbled feta cheese
- 1 ½ minced garlic clove
- 1 ½ tablespoon all-purpose flour
- black pepper house - made ground

Directions:

1. Preheat the oven to 425°F.
2. Line a pie pan with the piecrust and use a fork to pierce the crust in several places.
3. Bake the crust for 11 minutes. Remove from the oven and reduce the temperature to 325°F.
4. In a medium bowl, mix the broccoli, tomato, scallions, eggs, basil, rice milk, feta, garlic, and flour.
5. Season with pepper.
6. Pour the broccoli-and-egg mixture into the prepared pie pan.
7. Bake for 35 to 45 minutes, until a knife inserted in the center comes out clean.
8. Let cool for 12 to 15 minutes before serving.

Nutrition: Calories:160, Potassium:173 mg, Phosphorous: 101mg, Protein:6g, Sodium:259 mg, Fat:10g

ASPARAGUS FRITTATA

PREPARATION: 5 min.
COOKING TIME: 30 min.
SERVING: 2 People

Ingredients:

- 10 medium asparagus spears, ends trimmed
- 2 teaspoons extra-virgin olive oil, divided
- Freshly ground black pepper
- 4 large eggs
- ½ teaspoon onion powder
- ¼ cup chopped parsley

Directions:

1. Preheat the oven to 450°F.
2. Pour 1 teaspoon of olive oil into the asparagus and season with pepper.
3. Transfer to a baking pan and roast.
4. Stirring occasionally, for 25 minutes, until the spears are browned and tender.
5. In a small bowl, beat the eggs with the onion powder and parsley. Season with pepper.
6. Cut the asparagus spears into 1-inch pieces and arrange in a medium skillet.
7. Drizzle with the remaining oil and shake the pan to distribute.
8. Pour the egg mixture into the skillet and cook over medium heat. When the egg is well set on the bottom and nearly set on the top, cover it with a plate, invert the pan so the frittata is on the plate, and then slide it back into the pan with the cooked side up.
9. Continue to cook for about 35 more seconds, until firm.

Nutrition: Calories:102, Potassium:248 mg, Phosphorous: 103mg, Protein:6g, Sodium:46mg, Fat:8g

POACHED EGGS WITH CILANTRO BUTTER

PREPARATION: 5 min.
COOKING TIME: 10 min.
SERVING: 2 People

Ingredients:
- 2 tablespoons unsalted butter
- 1 tablespoon chopped parsley
- 1 tablespoon chopped cilantro
- 4/5 large eggs
- Dash vinegar
- Freshly ground black pepper

Directions:
1. In a small pan over low heat, melt the butter. Add the parsley and cilantro, and cook for about 2 minute, stirring constantly.
2. Remove from the heat and pour into a small dish.
3. In a small saucepan, bring about 3 ½ inches of water to a simmer.
4. Add the dash of vinegar.
5. Crack 1 egg into a cup or ramekin. Using a spoon, create a whirlpool in the simmering water, and then pour the egg into the water. Use the spoon to draw the white together until just starting to set.
6. Repeat with the remaining eggs.
7. Cook for 5 to 7 minutes, depending on how set you like your yolk.
8. With a slotted spoon, remove the eggs.
9. Serve the eggs topped with 1 tablespoon of the herbed butter and some pepper.

Nutrition: Calories:261, Potassium:173 mg, Phosphorous:226mg ,Protein:14g, Sodium:164mg, Fat:7g

GREEN BREAKFAST SOUP

PREPARATION: 5 min.
COOKING TIME: 5 min.
SERVING: 2 People

Ingredients:
- 2 cups spinach
- 2 cups low-sodium vegetable or chicken broth (see Lower sodium tip)
- 1 teaspoon ground coriander
- 1 teaspoon ground cumin
- 1 teaspoon ground turmeric
- Freshly ground black pepper

Directions:
1. In a blender or food processor, add the spinach, broth, coriander, cumin, and turmeric. Process until smooth.
2. Transfer the mixture to a small saucepan over medium heat, and cook until heated through, 2 to 3 minutes. Season with pepper.

Nutrition: Calories:221, Potassium:551mg, Phosphorous:58mg, Protein:5g Sodium:170 mg, Fat:18g

TASTY PANCAKES

PREPARATION: 15 min.
COOKING TIME: 12 min.
SERVING: 4 People

Ingredients:
- 1 cup all-purpose flour
- ½ cup sugar
- ½ teaspoon phosphorus-free baking powder
- 1 cup homemade rice milk
- 2 eggs
- 1 tablespoon unsalted butter

Directions:
1. Add the flour, sugar, and baking powder in a medium bowl. Stir well.
2. In a separate bowl, whisk together the rice milk and eggs.
3. Add the milk mixture to the flour mixture. Beat until incorporated.
4. Melt half of the butter in a pan over medium heat.
5. Spread the batter, about ¼ cup for each pancake, into the pan.
6. Cook the pancakes part by part about 3 minutes, until the edges are firm, and the bottoms are golden.
7. Repeat with the remaining butter and batter.
8. Serve hot and enjoy!

Nutrition: Calories:284, Potassium:113 mg, Phosphorous: 114mg, Protein:7g, Sodium:40mg, Fat:6g

SLOW COOKED OATS

PREPARATION: 5 min.
COOKING TIME: 30 min.
SERVING: 9 People

Ingredients:
- 1 tablespoon non-dairy butter substitute
- 1 cup steel cut oats
- 2 cups non-dairy milk
- 1 ½ cup water
- 2 teaspoons vanilla extract
- 1 tablespoon pure maple syrup
- ¼ cup and 2 tablespoons unsweetened peanut butter
- 1 ½ cups fresh blueberries

Directions:
1. Heat oil in a pan over medium heat.
2. Add the oats, stir frequently and toast for 3 minutes.
3. Add the milk, water and vanilla to boil increasing to medium-high heat.
4. Stir well.
5. Cover and cook 20-30 minutes with low simmer heat.
6. Stir from time to time.
7. Add the maple syrup and peanut butter.
8. Stir to combine.
9. Place in serving bowls and decorate with blueberries.
10. Serve and enjoy!

Nutrition: Calories:242, Potassium:205 mg, Phosphorous:59mg, Protein:7g Sodium:112mg, Fat:12g

PAPAYA ORANGE SMOOTHIE

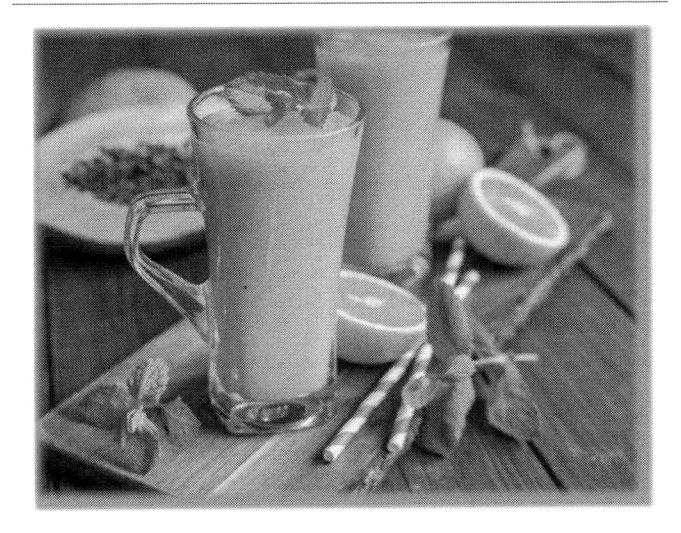

PREPARATION: 5 min.
COOKING TIME: 2 min.
SERVING: 1 Person

Ingredients:
- 3-ounces papaya, cut in small pieces
- ½ cup unsweetened almond milk
- 1 teaspoon honey
- ½ teaspoon fresh ginger, grated
- 2 tablespoons lime juice
- 2 ice cubes

Directions:
1. Add the papaya, milk, honey, ginger and lime in the blender.
2. Blend on medium speed for 15 seconds and add the ice cubes.
3. Blend on high speed about 30 seconds until smooth.
4. Serve and enjoy!

Nutrition: Calories:85, Potassium:276 mg, Phosphorous:25mg, Protein:1g, Sodium:94mg, Fat:2g

BROWN MUFFINS

PREPARATION: 15 min.
COOKING TIME: 30 min.
SERVING: 18 People

Ingredients:
- Cooking spray
- ½ cup buckwheat flour
- ¾ cup almond flour
- 1 cup unbleached all-purpose flour
- 6 tablespoons cocoa powder
- 1 teaspoon baking powder
- ½ teaspoon sea salt
- 1/2 cup light brown sugar
- 1/33 cup sunflower or other vegetable oil
- 2 large eggs
- 1 teaspoon pure vanilla extract
- ½ cup whole milk yogurt
- 4 large (6-ounce) medjool dates, pitted, diced
- 1/3 cup roasted pumpkin seeds

Directions:
1. Preheat oven to 350° F.
2. Spray a muffin tray with cooking spray and set aside. Arrange for 18 muffins.
3. In a large bowl pour dry ingredients and whisk well. Set aside.
4. In a separate bowl beat with the electric mixer the sugar and oil until fluffy.
5. Add the eggs, one at a time beating until well included.
6. Add the vanilla, and yogurt. Stir until well incorporated.
7. Add slowly the dry components. Mix until combined well.

8. Add the diced dates and pumpkin seeds. Mix well.
9. Spoon into a muffin tray and bake for about 25 minutes.
10. Serve warm and enjoy!

Nutrition: Calories:185, Potassium:249 mg, Phosphorous:112mg, Protein:5g, Sodium:106mg, Fat:10g

EASY CORN PUDDING

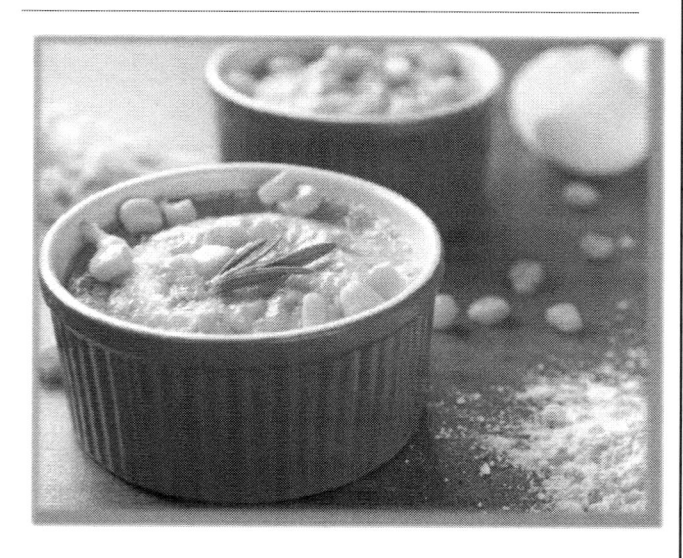

PREPARATION: 10 min.
COOKING TIME: 40 min.
SERVING: 7 People

Ingredients:

- Non-salted butter, for greasing the baking dish
- ¾ cup unsweetened rice milk, at room temperature
- 2 tablespoons light sour cream
- 2 tablespoons all-purpose flour
- ½ teaspoon Ener-G® Baking Soda baking soda substitute
- 3-4 eggs
- 3 tablespoons unsalted butter, melted
- 2 tablespoons caster sugar
- 2 cups defrost frozen corn kernels

Directions:

1. Preheat the oven to 350°F.
2. Grease a baking dish with butter and set aside.
3. In a mixing bowl add the flour and baking soda substitute. Stir well and set aside.
4. In a separate bowl, whisk the eggs, rice milk, butter, sour cream and sugar.
5. Blend the two mixtures together until smooth.
6. Add the corn to the batter. Stir until well mixed.
7. Bake for about 45 minutes after spooning the batter into the pan.
8. Let the pudding cool for about 18 minutes.
9. Serve warm and enjoy!

Nutrition: Calories:182, Potassium:199 mg, Phosphorous:116mg, Protein:6g, Sodium:62mg, Fat:12g

SLICED APPLE COOKIES

PREPARATION: 5 min.
COOKING TIME: -
SERVING: 8 People

Ingredients:

- 1 large coreless apple
- 2 tablespoons almond butter
- 1/3 cup muesli
- ¼ cup fresh blueberries

Directions:

1. Slice apple horizontally into about 8 rings.
2. Sprawl some almond butter on every apple ring.
3. Sprinkle the muesli on top and add the blueberries.
4. Serve and enjoy!

Nutrition: Calories:134, Potassium:180 mg, Phosphorous:92mg, Protein:4g, Sodium:4mg, Fat:7g

CHOCOLATE MUFFINS

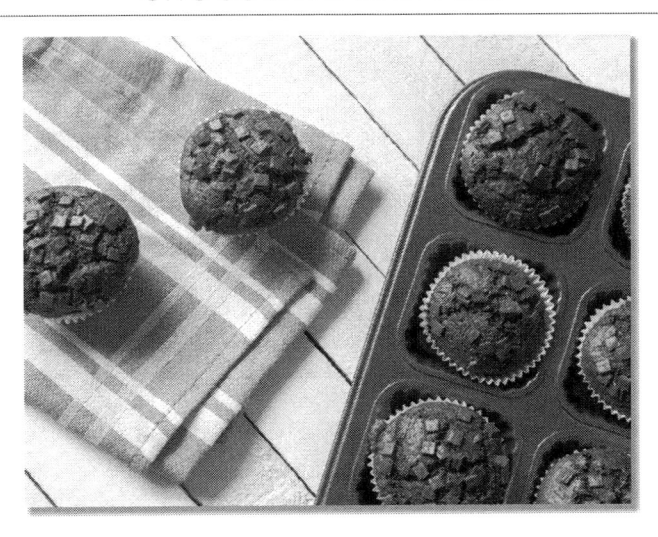

PREPARATION: 20 min.
COOKING TIME: 12 min.
SERVING: 12 People

Ingredients:

- 1 large egg
- 1/3 cup light brown sugar
- 1/4 cup olive oil
- 2 tablespoons plain yogurt
- 1 teaspoon vanilla extract
- 1 cup unbleached, all-purpose flour
- ¼ teaspoon sea salt
- ½ teaspoon baking soda
- ¼ teaspoon nutmeg
- 1/3 cup almonds, sliced
- 2/3 cup dark chocolate chips

Directions:

1. Preheat the oven to 350°F.
2. Spray a muffin tray with cooking spray and set aside.
3. In a mixing bowl add egg, sugar and oil and stir well.

4. Add yogurt and vanilla and mix with fork until smooth.
5. Add the flour ¼ cup at a time, with salt and baking soda in between additions.
6. Stir well.
7. Combine almonds and chocolate chips.
8. Bake for about 12 minutes.
9. Serve and enjoy!

Nutrition: Calories:148, Potassium:140 mg Phosphorous: 45mg, Protein:3g, Sodium:111mg, Fat:7g

SAVORY SPRING MUFFINS

PREPARATION: 12 min.
COOKING TIME: 10 min.
SERVING: 30 People

Ingredients:

- 1 tablespoon olive oil
- 1 cup red bell pepper, chopped
- 1 green bell pepper, chopped
- 1 cup onion, chopped
- 2 cup spinach, chopped
- 2 cloves of garlic
- 1 cup mushrooms, chopped
- 4 eggs

Directions:

1. Preheat oven to 350°F.
2. Heat oil in a pan.
3. Add peppers, onion and cook until tender.
4. Add spinach, garlic and mushrooms and cook for 2 more minutes.
5. In a mixing bowl add the eggs and blend together.
6. Stir in cooked vegetables.
7. Spread the batter into the muffing tray.
8. Bake for about 20 minutes.
9. Serve and enjoy!

Nutrition: Calories:54, Potassium:147 mg, Phosphorous:57mg, Protein:4g, Sodium:38mg, Fat:0g

PITA WITH EGG & CURRY

PREPARATION: 18 min.
COOKING TIME: 5 min.
SERVING: 4 People

Ingredients:

- 3 eggs, beaten
- 1 scallion, chopped
- ½ red bell pepper, chopped
- 2 teaspoons unsalted butter
- 1 teaspoon curry powder
- ½ teaspoon ground ginger
- 2 tablespoons light sour cream
- 2 (4-inch) plain pita bread pockets, halved
- ½ cup English cucumber, julienned
- 1 cup watercress, chopped

Directions:

1. In a mixing bowl add the eggs, scallion, and red pepper. Whisk together until well combined.
2. Melt the butter in a nonstick pan over medium heat.
3. Pour the egg mixture into the pan and cook for about 3 minutes, swirling the skillet but not stirring. Set aside.

4. In a mixing bowl, stir the curry powder, ginger, and sour cream until well mixed.
5. Evenly divide the curry sauce among the 4 halves of the pita bread, spreading it out on one inside edge.
6. Split the cucumber and watercress evenly between the halves.
7. Split the eggs into the halves.
8. Serve and enjoy!

Nutrition: Calories:126, Potassium:166 mg, Phosphorous: 108mg, Protein:8g, Sodium:138mg, Fat:7g

HOT VANILLA CEREALS

PREPARATION: 10 min.
COOKING TIME: 25 min.
SERVING: 4 People

Ingredients:

- 2¼ cups water
- 1¼ cups vanilla rice milk
- 6 tablespoons uncooked bulgur
- 2 tablespoons uncooked whole buckwheat
- 1 cup apple, peeled and sliced
- 6 tablespoons plain uncooked couscous
- ½ teaspoon ground cinnamon

Directions:

1. Heat the water and the rice milk in a pan over medium-high heat.
2. Bring to a boil, and add the bulgur, buckwheat, and apple.
3. Cook for about 25 minutes over low heat, stirring occasionally.
4. Remove the saucepan from the heat and stir in the couscous and cinnamon.
5. Let the saucepan stand, covered, for 10 minutes.
6. Serve and enjoy!

Nutrition: Calories:172, Potassium:141 mg, Phosphorous:132mg, Protein:4g, Sodium:34mg, Fat:1g

AROMATIC CARROT CREAM

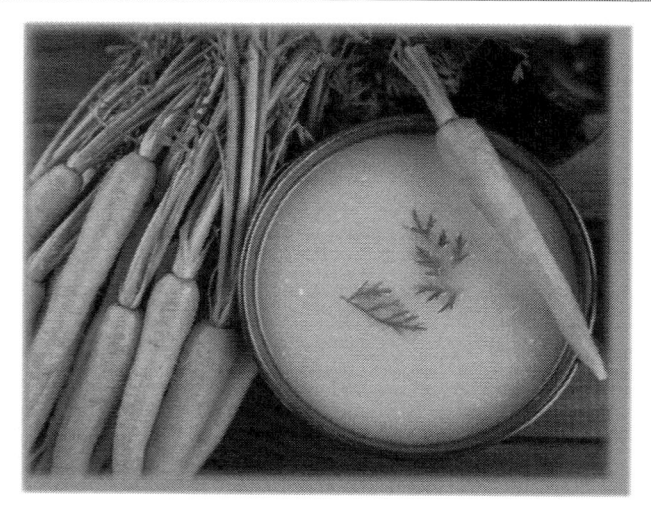

PREPARATION: 15 min.
COOKING TIME: 25 min.
SERVING: 4 People

Ingredients:

- 1 tablespoon olive oil
- ½ sweet onion, chopped
- 2 teaspoons fresh ginger, peeled and grated
- 1 teaspoon fresh garlic, minced
- 4 cups water
- 3 carrots, chopped
- 1 teaspoon ground turmeric
- ½ cup coconut milk

Directions:

1. Heat the olive oil into a big pan over medium-high heat.
2. Add the onion, garlic and ginger. Softly cook for about 3 minutes until softened.
3. Include the water, turmeric and the carrots. Softly cook for about 20 minutes (until the carrots are softened).
4. Blend the soup adding coconut milk until creamy.
5. Serve and enjoy!

Nutrition: Calories:112, Potassium:241 mg, Phosphorous:59mg, Protein:2g, Sodium:35mg, Fat:10g

MUSHROOMS VELVET SOUP

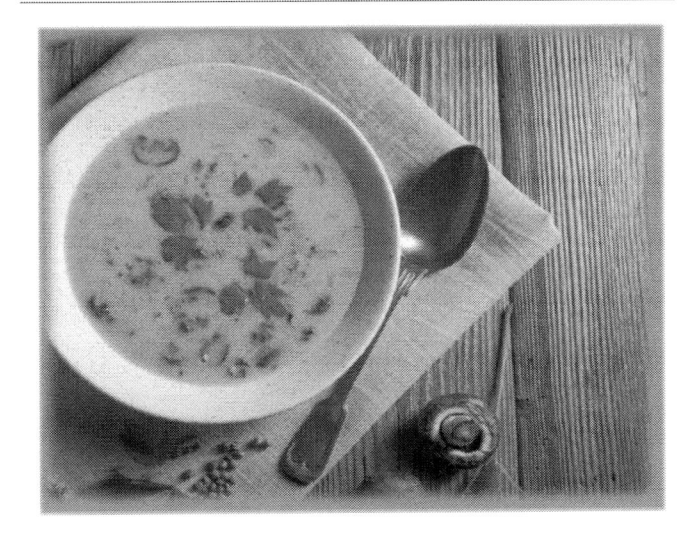

PREPARATION: 40 min.
COOKING TIME: 40 min.
SERVING: 6 People

Ingredients:

- 1 teaspoon olive oil
- ½ teaspoon fresh ground black pepper
- 3 medium (85g) shallots, diced
- 2 stalks (80g) celery, chopped
- 1 clove garlic, diced
- 12-ounces cremini mushrooms, sliced
- 5 tablespoons flour
- 4 cups low sodium vegetable stock, divided
- 3 sprigs fresh thyme
- 2 bay leaves
- ½ cup regular yogurt

Directions:

1. Heat oil in a large pan.
2. Add ground pepper, shallots and celery. Cook over medium-high heat.
3. Sauté for 2 minutes until golden.
4. Add garlic and stir over medium heat for about 2 minutes.
5. Include the sliced mushrooms. Stir and cook for 12 minutes until the mushrooms release their liquid.
6. Sprawl the flour on the mushrooms and toast for about 3 minutes.
7. Add one cup of hot stock, thyme sprigs and bay leaves.
8. Stir and add the second cup of stock. Stir until well combined.
9. Add the remaining cups of broth.
10. Slowly cook for 15 minutes.
11. Take out thyme sprigs and bay leaves.
12. Blend with an immersion blender until mixture is smooth.
13. Include the yogurt and stir well.
14. Slowly cook for 4 minutes.
15. Serve and enjoy!

Nutrition: Calories:126, Potassium:298 mg, Phosphorous:70mg, Protein:3g, Sodium:108mg, Fat:8g

EASY LETTUCE WRAPS

PREPARATION: 15 min.
COOKING TIME: - min.
SERVING: 4 People

Ingredients:

- 8 ounces cooked chicken, shredded
- 1 scallion, chopped
- ½ cup seedless red grapes, halved
- 1 celery stalk, chopped
- 1/4 cup mayonnaise
- A pinch ground black pepper
- 4 large lettuce leaves

Directions:

1. In a mixing bowl add the scallion, chicken, celery, grapes and mayonnaise.
2. Stir well until incorporated.
3. Season with pepper.
4. Place the lettuce leaves onto serving plates.
5. Place the chicken salad onto the leaves.
6. Serve and enjoy!

Nutrition: Calories:146, Potassium:212 mg, Phosphorous:125mg, Protein:16g, Sodium:58mg, Fat:5g

SPAGHETTI WITH PESTO

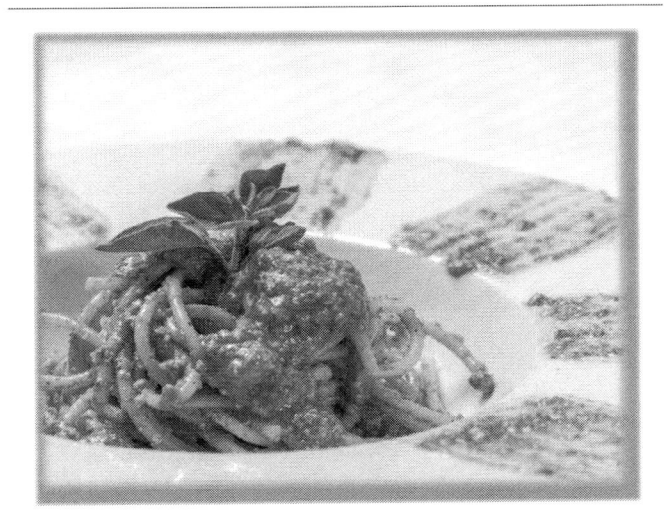

PREPARATION: 10 min.
COOKING TIME: 10 min.
SERVING: 4 People

Ingredients:

- 8 ounces spaghetti (package pasta)
- 2 cups packed basil leaves
- 2 cups packed arugula leaves
- 1/3 cup walnut pieces
- 3 cloves of garlic
- ¼ cup extra-virgin olive oil
- Black pepper

Directions:

1. Cook pasta in a large pot of boiling water until done. Drain.
2. Add the basil, garlic, olive oil, walnuts, pepper and arugula in a blender and mix until creamy.
3. In a large bowl, mix pesto mixture into pasta.
4. Serve and enjoy!

Nutrition: Calories:400, Potassium:202 mg, Phosphorous:113mg, Protein:11g, Sodium:6mg, Fat:21g

SPICED WRAPS

PREPARATION: 10 min.
COOKING TIME: - min.
SERVING: 8 People

Ingredients:

- 6 ounces cooked chicken breast, minced
- 1 scallion, chopped
- ½ red apple, cored and chopped
- ½ cup bean sprouts
- ¼ cucumber, chopped
- Juice of 1 lime
- Zest of 1 lime
- 2 tablespoons fresh cilantro, chopped
- ½ teaspoon Chinese five-spice powder
- 8 lettuce leaves

Directions:

1. In a mixing bowl combine the chicken, apple, bean sprouts, cucumber, lime juice, lime zest, cilantro, five-spice powder and scallions.
2. Place the lettuce leaves onto 8 serving plates.
3. Spoon the chicken mixture onto lettuce leaves.
4. Wrap the lettuce around the chicken mixture.
5. Serve and enjoy!

Nutrition: Calories:53 Potassium:134mg, Phosphorous:58mg, Protein:7g, Sodium:19mg, Fat:3g

POACHED ASPARAGUS AND EGG

PREPARATION: 3 min.
COOKING TIME: 15min.
SERVING: 4 People 1

Ingredients:
- 1 egg
- 4 spears asparagus
- Water

Directions:
1. Half-fill a deep saucepan with water set over high heat. Let the water come to a boil.
2. Dip asparagus spears in water. Cook until they turn a shade brighter, about 3 minutes. Remove from saucepan and drain on paper towels. Keep warm. Lightly season prior to serving.
3. Using a slotted spoon, gently lower egg into boiling water. Cook for only 4 minutes. Remove from pan immediately. Place on egg holder.
4. Slice off the top. The egg should still be fluid inside.
5. Place asparagus spears on a small plate and serve egg on the side. Dip asparagus into the egg and eat while warm.

Nutrition: Calories 178, Carbs 1g, Fat 13g, Protein 7.72g, Potassium (K) 203 mg, Sodium (Na) 71 mg, Phosphorus 124 mg

APPLE TURNOVER

PREPARATION: 10 min.
COOKING TIME: 15 min.
SERVING: 8 People

Ingredients:

For the turnovers:
- ½ tsp. cinnamon powder
- All-purpose flour
- ½ cup unwashed palm sugar
- 1 tbsp. almond flour
- 4 peeled, cored and diced baking apples.

For the egg wash:
- 2 tbsps. water
- 1 whisked egg white

Directions:
1. To make the filling: combine almond flour, cinnamon powder and palm sugar until these resemble coarse meal. Toss in diced apples until well coated. Set aside.
2. On a lightly floured surface, roll out the puff pastry until ¼ inch thin.
3. Slice into 8 pieces of 4"x 4" squares.
4. Divide the prepared apples into 8 equal portions. Spoon on individual puff pastry squares. Fold in half diagonally. Press edges to seal.
5. Place each filled pastry on a baking tray lined with parchment paper. Make sure there is ample space between pastries.

6. Freeze for at least 25 minutes, or until ready to bake.
7. Preheat oven to 400°F for 12 minutes.
8. Brush frozen pastries with egg wash. Place in the hot oven, and cook for 12 to 15 minutes, or until they turn golden brown all over.
9. Remove baking tray from oven immediately.
10. Cool slightly for easier handling.
11. Place 1 apple turnover on a plate. Serve warm.

Nutrition: Protein 3.81g, Potassium (K) 151 mg, Sodium (Na) 86 mg, Carbs 35.75g, Calories 285, Fat 14.78g, Phosphorus 43.4mg

EGG DROP SOUP

PREPARATION: 5 min.
COOKING TIME: 10 min.
SERVING: 4 People

Ingredients:
- ¼ cup minced fresh chives
- 4 cups unsalted vegetable stock
- 4 whisked eggs

Directions:
1. Pour unsalted vegetable stock into the oven set over high heat. Bring to a boil. Turn down heat to the lowest heat setting.
2. Pour in the eggs. Stir continuously until ribbons form into the soup.
3. Turn off the heat immediately. The residual heat will cook eggs through.
4. Cool slightly before ladling the desired amount into individual bowls.
5. Garnish with a pinch of parsley, if using. Serve immediately.

Nutrition: Calories 32, Carbs 0g, Fat 2 g, Protein 5.57g, Potassium (K) 67 mg, Sodium (Na) 63 mg, Phosphorus 36.1mg

ROASTED PEPPER SOUP

PREPARATION: 10 min.
COOKING TIME: 30 min.
SERVING: 4 People

Ingredients:
- 2 cups unsalted vegetable broth
- ½ cup chopped carrots
- 2 large red peppers
- ¼ cup julienned sweet basil
- 2 minced garlic cloves
- ½ cup chopped celery
- 2 tbsps. Olive oil
- ½ cup chopped onion
- ½ cup almond milk

Directions:
1. Place the oven into the 375°F.
2. Put onions on a baking sheet. Add the red peppers beside the mixture. Drizzle some of the olive oil over everything and toss well to coat.
3. Roast for 20 minutes, or until peppers are tender and skins are wilted.
4. Chop the roasted red peppers and set aside.

5. Place a pot over medium high flame and heat through. Once hot, add the olive oil and swirl to coat.
6. Place the carrot, celery, and garlic into the pot and sauté until carrot and celery are tender. Add the chopped roasted red peppers. Mix well.
7. Pour in the vegetable broth and almond milk. Increase to high flame and bring to a boil.
8. Once boiling, reduce to a simmer. Simmer, uncovered, for 10 minutes.
9. Turn off the heat and allow to cool slightly.
10. If desired, blend the soup using an immersion blender until the soup has reached a desired level of smoothness. Reheat over medium flame.
11. Add the basil and stir to combine.
12. Serve.

Nutrition: Calories 320, Protein 1.3g, Potassium (K) 249 mg, Sodium (Na) 45 mg Fat 25g, Carbs 20g, Phosphorus 66.33 g

ASSORTED FRESH FRUIT JUICE

PREPARATION: 5 min.
COOKING TIME: 0 min.
SERVING: 1 Person

Ingredients:
- 1 roughly chopped apple
- ¼ cup halved frozen grapes
- 1 cup ice shavings

Directions:
1. Add all ingredients into the blender.
2. Process until smooth.
3. Pour equal portions into glasses. Serve immediately.

Nutrition: Calories 112, Protein 1.16g, Potassium (K) 367 mg, Sodium (Na) 3 mg, Fat 0.5g, Carbs 25.8g Phosphorus 17.4mg

RASPBERRY AND PINEAPPLE SMOOTHIE

PREPARATION: 5 min.
COOKING TIME: 5 min.
SERVING: 4 People

Ingredients:

- ½ cup crushed ice
- 8 oz. rinsed and drained pineapple tidbits
- ½ cup frozen raspberries

Direction:

1. Except for cashew nuts and stevia, combine remaining ingredients in a deep microwave-safe bowl. Stir.
2. Microwave on the highest setting for 5 to 15 seconds. Keep a watchful eye on this. Stop the cooking process before milk bubbles out of the bowl.
3. Carefully remove the bowl from microwave. Cool slightly for easier handling.
4. Stir in stevia if using. Sprinkle cashew nuts.

Nutrition: Protein 3.1g, Potassium (K) 749 mg, Sodium (Na) 4 mg, Calories 360, Fat 1g, Carbs 90g, Phosphorus 106.2mg

MEXICAN FRITTATA

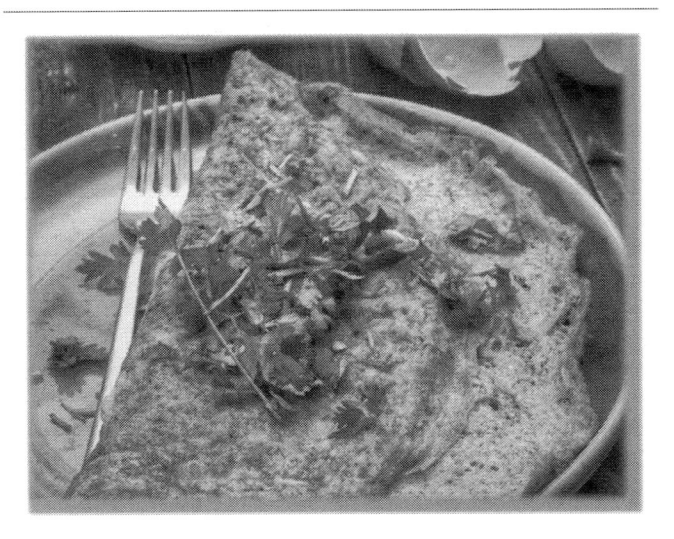

PREPARATION: 5 min.
COOKING TIME: 20 min.
SERVING: 2 People

Ingredients:

- 5 large eggs
- ¼ cup chopped green bell pepper
- ¼ cup chopped onions
- ½ cup almond milk

Direction:

1. Preheat the oven to 400° F.
2. Using a large bowl, combine almond milk, eggs, onion, and green bell pepper. Whisk until all ingredients are well combined.
3. Transfer the mixture to a baking dish. Bake for 20 minutes. Serve.

Nutrition: Calories 239.5, Protein 16.35g, Potassium (K) 243 mg, Sodium (Na) 216 mg, Carbs 5.3 g, Fat 17.0 g, Phosphorus 94 mg

OLIVE OIL AND SESAME ASPARAGUS

PREPARATION: 5 min.
COOKING TIME: 5 min.
SERVING: 1 Person

Ingredients:

- ½ tbsp. olive oil
- 2 cups sliced asparagus
- ½ cup water
- ½ tsp. sesame seeds
- 1/8 tsp. crushed red pepper flakes

Direction:

1. In a large skillet, bring water to a boil.
2. Add in asparagus. Allow to boil for 2 minutes. Reduce the heat and cook for another 5 minutes. Drain asparagus and place on a plate. Set aside.
3. Meanwhile, heat the olive oil. Tip in asparagus and red pepper flakes. Sauté for 3 minutes.
4. Remove from heat. Drizzle in more olive oil and sprinkle sesame seeds before serving.

Nutrition: Calories 122, Protein 6.19g, Potassium (K) 547 mg, Sodium (Na) 9 mg Fat 7g, Carbs 11g, Phosphorus:37mg

BREAKFAST CHEESECAKE

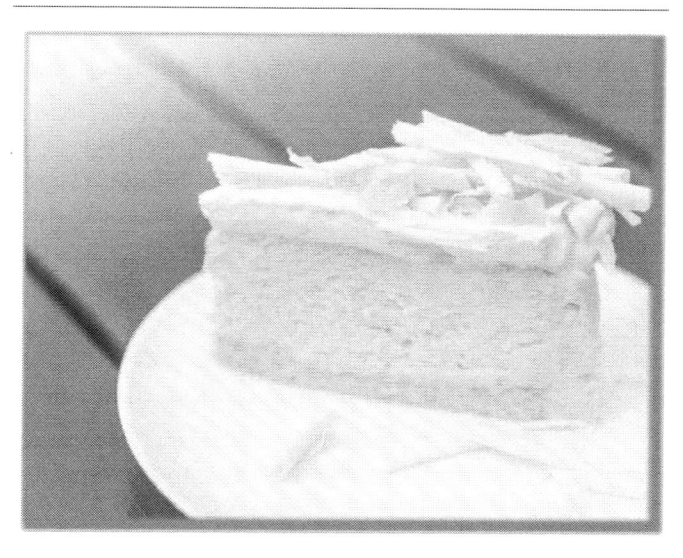

PREPARATION: 5 min.
COOKING TIME: 15 min.
SERVING: 16 People

Ingredients:

- ½ cup uncured sausage
- 2 tbsps. honey
- 7 cups cottage cheese
- Pepper, ¼ tsp.
- ½ tsp. olive oil
- 7 cups Greek yogurt
- Salt, ¼ tsp.
- 4 eggs
- 2 tsps. vanilla
- ½ chopped onion

Direction:

1. In a blender, combine eggs, cream cheese, cottage cheese, honey, and vanilla. Process until all ingredients are well combined.
2. Meanwhile, heat the olive oil in a pan. Sauté onion and uncured sausage. Season with salt and pepper. Cook for 4 minutes. Transfer the mixture into a baking dish.
3. Place inside the oven and bake for 10 minutes. Allow to cool at room temperature. Refrigerate for 1 hour before serving.

Nutrition: Protein 22.92g, Potassium (K) 244 mg, Sodium (Na) 477 mg, Phosphorus 106mg, Carbs 8.1g, Fat 6.1g, Calories 121.3

EGGS CREAMY MELT

PREPARATION: 6 min.
COOKING TIME: 4 min.
SERVING: 2 People

Ingredients:

- 1 tbsp. olive oil
- Italian seasoning
- 1 cup shredded tofu
- 2 beaten eggs

Direction:

1. In a small bowl, combine beaten eggs and Italian seasoning. Sprinkle tofu on top.
2. Heat the olive oil in a pan. Add the egg mixture. Cook for 4 minutes on both sides. Serve.

Nutrition: Protein 15.57g, Potassium (K) 216 mg, Sodium (Na) 107 mg, Calories 214, Fat 16.9 g, Carbs 1.4 g Phosphorous 73 mg

STUFFED CRIMINI MUSHROOMS WITH BASIL PESTO

PREPARATION: 12 min.
COOKING TIME: 15 min.
SERVING: 20 People

Ingredients:

- 20 crimini mushrooms, stems trimmed and rinsed
- 2 c basil leaves, fresh
- 2 teaspoons pumpkin seeds
- 1/4 cup fresh Parmesan
- 1 teaspoon of extra virgin olive oil
- lemon juice (2 teaspoons)
- kosher salt (half teaspoon)
- fresh garlic, 1 tbsp
- 1 ½ cups breadcrumbs (panko)
- 1 ½ tablespoon melted butter
- 2 tbsp. fresh parsley, chopped

Directions:

1. Preheat the oven to 350 degrees F.
2. Place the mushroom caps on a baking pan upside down.
3. To make the topping, mix the panko, butter, and parsley in a small dish and put it aside.
4. Place the basil, cheese, pumpkin seeds, oil, garlic, lemon juice, and salt in a food processor to make the filling. Mix until everything is well combined.
5. Fill the mushroom caps generously with the basil pesto filling.
6. 1 teaspoon panko topping on each mushroom
7. Gently rub the topping down. Preheat the oven to 350°F and bake for 13 to 15 minutes, or until golden brown.

Nutrition: Calories: 60 Protein:1,9g; Sodium:78 mg; Fat:3,5g

DILLY SCRAMBLED EGGS WITH GOAT CHEESE

PREPARATION: 5 min.
COOKING TIME: 5 min.
SERVING: 2 People

Ingredients:

- 2 large eggs
- 1 teaspoon dried dill weed
- 1 tablespoon crumbled goat cheese
- 1/8 teaspoon black pepper

Directions:

- In a mixing bowl, whisk together the eggs; pour into a nonstick skillet over medium heat.
- Toss the eggs with black pepper and dill.
- Scramble the eggs in the pan.
- Before serving, sprinkle the top with crumbled goat cheese.

Nutrition: Calories: 197; Protein:15 g; Carbs: 1,2g; Sodium:211 mg; Potassium: 190 mg; Fat:13g; Calcium: 212 mg

REDUCED-FAT BREAKFAST CASSEROLE

PREPARATION: 5 min.
COOKING TIME: 5 min.
SERVING: 8 People

Ingredients:

- 4 large eggs
- 1/2 teaspoon dry mustard
- 7 ounces reduced-fat pork sausage
- 1 cup 1% low-fat milk
- 8 ounces cream cheese
- 1/2 teaspoon dried onion flakes
- 3 slices white bread, cubed or broken

Directions:

1. Preheat the oven to 325 degrees Fahrenheit.
2. In a medium pan, crumble sausage and cook until done; put aside.
3. In a blender, combine the remaining ingredients, except the bread.
4. Toss in the cooked sausage with the rest of the ingredients.
5. Fill a greased 9" × 9" casserole dish partially with bread pieces.
6. Pour the sausage mixture on top of the bread.
7. Preheat oven to 350°F and bake for 55 minutes, or until set.
8. Cut the pie into 8 pieces and serve.

Nutrition: Calories: 220; Protein:9,5; Carbs: 7g; Sodium:320 mg; Potassium 190 mg; Fat:13g.

BREAKFAST CEREAL MIX

PREPARATION: 5 min.
COOKING TIME: 0 min.
SERVING: 5 People

Ingredients:

- 1/2 cup Cocoa Puffs® cereal
- 1/2 cup mini rice cakes
- 1 cup Rice Chex® cereal
- 1 cup Corn Chex® cereal

Directions:

- Combine all ingredients in a medium mixing basin.
- Divide the mixture into 1 cup parts.
- Serve dry or with a milk alternative of your choice.

Nutrition: Calories: 143 Protein:0,8 g; Carbs: 31 g; Sodium:233 mg; Potassium 69 mg; Fat:0,9 g; Calcium 94g

FRENCH TOAST WITH TASTY STRAWBERRY CREAM CHEESE

PREPARATION: 5 min.
COOKING TIME: 5 min.
SERVING: 10 People

Ingredients:

- 10 slices Texas toast-style bread
- 1/3 cup maple syrup
- 2 teaspoons unsalted butter
- 11 ounces cold cream cheese
- 1-1/2 cups half & half creamer
- 2 cups fresh strawberries
- 8 large eggs
- 3 cups white granulated sugar

Directions:

1. Coat a 9 x 13-inch baking dish thoroughly with nonstick cooking spray.
2. Cut the bread and cream cheese into cubes. Slice the strawberries into two 1-cup chunks, one of which will be kept aside. Half of the bread cubes should be placed in the prepared dish. Over the top of the bread, layer the cream cheese cubes. One cup cut strawberries on top of cream cheese, followed by the remaining bread pieces.
3. Whisk together eggs, half-and-half, and maple syrup in a large mixing basin until thoroughly blended. Then, using a spatula, evenly distribute the mixture over the bread cubes.
4. To wet the bread entirely, gently press it with the back of a spoon. Refrigerate for at least 7/8 hours or overnight.
5. Preheat the oven to 350 degrees Fahrenheit.
6. Bake the pan uncovered for about 50 minutes, or until puffed and golden brown and a knife placed in the middle comes out clean.
7. While the dish is cooking, make the sauce. Toss the remaining 1 cup of strawberries with the sugar in a small bowl. Allow for 20 minutes of resting time, stirring periodically. Then, puree the mixture in a blender or food processor until smooth.
8. In a small saucepan, pour the strawberry sauce. Stir in the butter and cook for about 5 minutes over medium heat, stirring regularly.
9. Cool for 5 minutes after removing the dish from the oven. Serve with warm strawberry sauce and cut into 12 portions.

Nutrition: Calories: 335; Protein:10 g; Carbs: 39 g; Sodium:235 mg; Potassium 237 mg; Phosphorus 170; Fat:15 g; Calcium 149g

CREAM CHEESE GOLDEN BAGEL

PREPARATION: 5 min.
COOKING TIME: 5 min.
SERVING: 2 People

Ingredients:

- 1 bagel, 2-ounce size
- 2 tablespoons cream cheese
- 2 tomato slices, 1/4-inch thick
- 1 teaspoon low-sodium lemon pepper seasoning
- 2 red onion slices

Directions:

- Toast the bagel slices till golden brown.
- Spread cream cheese on both halves of the bagel.
- Sprinkle with lemon pepper and top with
- onion and tomato slices.

Nutrition: Calories: 133; Protein:4 g; Carbs: 18 g; Sodium:217 mg; Potassium 160 mg; Phosphorus 51; Fat:15 g; Calcium 8g

JAZZ APPLE OATMEAL

PREPARATION: 1min.
COOKING TIME: 5 min.
SERVING: 1 Person

Ingredients:

- 4 Jazz Apple or alternatively Pink Lady, peeled and split
- 2 tablespoons packed brown sugar
- ½ teaspoon ground cinnamon
- ¼ teaspoon salt
- 8 tbsp non-fat plain Greek yogurt
- 1 cup steel-cut oats
- 3/4 cups water

Directions:

1. Use the big holes of a box grater and shred two apples, leaving the core intact.
2. In a medium skillet, heat the oil over medium-high heat.
3. Cook, constantly stirring, until the oats are gently toasted, about 2-3 minutes.
4. Put the water and shredded apples to a boil.
5. Reduce heat to maintain a simmer and cook for 11 minutes, stirring constantly.
6. Chop the remaining two apples in the meantime.
7. Stir in the chopped apples, two tablespoons of brown sugar, cinnamon, and salt after the oats have steamed for 10-12 minutes; continue cooking, stirring periodically, until the apples are soft and the oatmeal is pretty thick, 15 to 20 minutes more.
8. Split the oatmeal into four bowls.
9. Put two tablespoons of yogurt and 3/4 teaspoon brown sugar on each portion.

Nutrition: Calories: 213; Protein:8 g; Sodium: 168 mg; Potassium 274 mg; Phosphorus 138; Fat:1.5 g; Calcium 70g

QUICK AND EASY COFFEE CUP EGG SCRAMBLE

PREPARATION: 5 min.
COOKING TIME: 5 min.
SERVING: 1 Person

Ingredients:

- 1 large egg
- 1/8 teaspoon black pepper
- 2 tablespoons 1% low fat milk
- 2 large egg whites

Directions:

1. Using cooking spray, coat a 12-ounce coffee cup. In a cup, whisk the milk, egg, and egg whites until smooth.
2. Cook for 30 - 60 seconds in a microwave-safe coffee cup; remove and stir. Microwave for another 30-45 seconds, or until the eggs are nearly set.
3. Enjoy with a pinch of black pepper.

Nutrition: Calories: 119; Protein:14 g; Carbs: 2,5 g; Sodium:194 mg; Potassium 224 mg; Phosphorus 137; Fat:4 g; Calcium 70g

PEPPERS AND ONIONS SCRAMBLED EGG WRAP

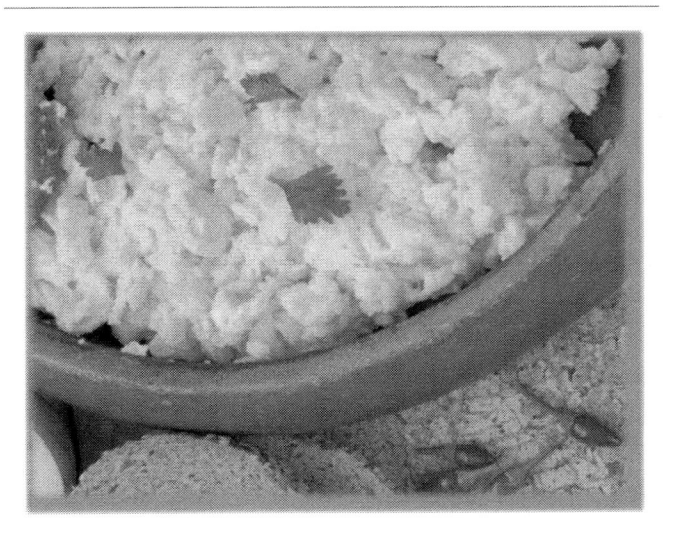

PREPARATION: 5 min.
COOKING TIME: 5 min.
SERVING: 1 Person

Ingredients:

- 3 eggs
- Pepper
- Salt-free seasoning
- Avocado oil cooking spray
- ¼ cup chopped bell pepper
- ¼ cup chopped onion
- 2 teaspoon chopped jalapeno

Directions:

1. In a large skillet, heat the oil over medium heat.
2. Apply cooking spray to the surface.
3. Mix in the peppers and onions.
4. Cook, occasionally stirring, until the onions begin to brown.
5. Eggs should be whisked.
6. Reduce the heat to medium-low and pour the eggs over the veggies.
7. Season with salt, pepper to taste.
8. Cook until the mixture is almost set.
9. Flip and cook until no liquid egg remains.

Nutrition: Calories: 205; Protein:14 g; Carbs: 5 g; Sodium:186 mg; Potassium 280 mg; Fat:12 g; Calcium 79g

REFRESHING AND TASTY SMOOTHIE

PREPARATION: 5 min.
COOKING TIME: 5 min.
SERVING: 1 Person

Ingredients:

- ½ cup frozen grapes
- 1 scoop chocolate whey protein powder
- ½ cup unsweetened almond milk

Directions:

1. Blend the frozen grapes in a blender.
2. Pour in almond milk (tip: search for one without "phosphate" additives on the ingredient line).
3. Add protein powder (whey is ideal; opt for one that is pure and free of additives).
4. Blend until completely smooth.

Nutrition: Calories:160; Protein:19 g; Carbs: 11 g; Sodium:119 mg; Potassium 337 mg; Fat:3,5 g; Calcium 227g

PROTEIN-PACKED TOFU SCRABLER

PREPARATION: 10 min.
COOKING TIME: 20 min.
SERVING: 2 People

Ingredients:

- ¼ cup green bell pepper, chopped
- 1 teaspoon olive oil
- ⅛ teaspoon turmeric
- ¼ teaspoon garlic powder
- 1 clove garlic, minced
- ¼ cup red bell pepper, chopped
- 1 cup firm tofu (choose less than 10% calcium)
- 1 teaspoon onion powder

Directions:

1. Sauté the garlic and bell peppers in olive oil in a medium-sized nonstick pan.
2. Toss the tofu into the skillet once it has been rinsed and drained.
3. Add the remaining components.
4. Cook at low to medium heat, occasionally stirring, for about 20 minutes, or until the tofu has turned a faint golden color. The moisture in the mixture will evaporate.
5. Tofu scrambler should be served warm.

Nutrition: Calories:160; Protein:19 g; Carbs: 11 g; Sodium:119 mg; Potassium 337 mg; Fat:3,5 g; Calcium 227g

60-SECONDS OMELETS WITH VEGGIES

PREPARATION: 1 min.
COOKING TIME: 1 min.
SERVING: 1 Person

Ingredients:
- 2 eggs (yolk included)
- 1/2 cup filling (vegetables, meat)
- 1 TBSP unsalted butter
- 2 TBSP water

Directions:
1. Blend eggs and water in a mixing bowl.
2. Melt butter in a small saucepan.
3. Fill the pan with the egg mixture.
4. The mixture should immediately solidify around the pan's edges.
5. Carefully push cooked omelet parts from the outer borders into the center with a spatula so the raw egg can fill the pan and cook.
6. Continue until the egg has set and is no longer flowing.
7. Fill one side of the omelet with 1/2 cup of your favorite filling.
8. Split the omelet in half with the spatula to complete cooking.

Nutrition: Calories:160; Protein:19 g; Carbs: 11 g; Sodium:119 mg; Potassium 337 mg; Fat:3,5 g; Calcium 227g

SAUSAGE BREAKFAST MUFFIN WITH EGG AND CHEESE

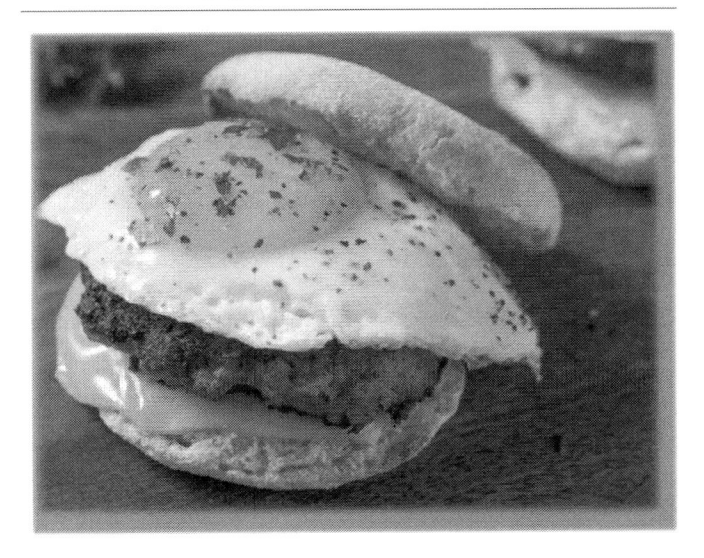

PREPARATION: 10 min.
COOKING TIME: 3 min.
SERVING: 1 Person

Ingredients:
- 1 tablespoon shredded natural sharp cheddar cheese
- nonstick frying spray
- 1/5 cup liquid low-cholesterol egg substitute
- 1 English muffin
- 1 turkey sausage patty

Directions:
1. Pour the egg product into a small pan prepared with nonstick cooking spray and cook over medium-low heat.
2. Once the egg is almost done, flip it with a spatula and cook again for 30 seconds.
3. Lightly toast an English muffin.
4. Place the turkey sausage patty on a platter, cover with a paper towel, and microwave for 1 minute, or until done according to package directions.

5. Place a cooked egg on top of an English muffin (fold to fit the muffin)—top with a sausage patty, then sharp cheddar cheese, then the other half of the muffin.

Nutrition: Calories:250; Protein:15 g; Carbs: 25 g; Sodium:589 mg; Potassium 215 mg; Fat:7 g; Calcium 170 g; Phosphorus 156 mg

HIGH-PROTEIN PEACH SMOOTHIE

PREPARATION: 10 min.
COOKING TIME: -
SERVING: 1 Person

Ingredients:

- 2 cup ice
- 1 tablespoon sugar
- 2 tablespoons egg whites
- 4 cup fresh peaches

Directions:

1. Mix the peaches until smooth in a blender.
2. Blend in the remaining ingredients until completely smooth.

Nutrition: Calories:129; Protein:11 g; Carbs: 22 g; Sodium:153 mg; Potassium 350 mg; Fat:0 g; Calcium 8 g; Phosphorus 35 mg

TASTY BREAKFAST TORTILLAS WITH RED HOT JALAPENO

PREPARATION: 12 min.
COOKING TIME: 10 min.
SERVING: 6 People

Ingredients:

- 3 cups pineapple, peeled and cut into 1/2" cubes
- 2 seeded and chopped jalapeno peppers
- 3 tbsp. roughly chopped fresh cilantro
- 6 x 10" flour tortillas
- 2 tbsp. lime juice
- 1 tsp. oil
- 1 tablespoon brown sugar (light brown)
- 12 giant eggs, beaten 1 cup diced green bell pepper 1 cup sliced and chopped shitake or button mushrooms
- pepper to taste, 1/4 cup green onion, chopped

Directions:

1. Prepare salsa, in a non-reactive bowl. (glass, ceramic, or ceramic).
2. Combine the pineapple, cilantro, jalapenos, lime juice, and brown sugar
3. Heat the oil in a nonstick pan and cook green peppers and mushrooms for about 5 minutes over medium heat.
4. Remove any extra liquid.
5. Pour the beaten eggs over the mixture in the skillet and equally sprinkle the green onion on top.
6. Spoon the eggs across the skillet with a spatula as they begin to solidify, generating big curds.
7. Cook and fold the eggs until there is no visible liquid egg left.
8. Season with salt and pepper.

9. Distribute the egg mixture evenly among the tortillas.
10. Fill each tortilla with 1/3 cup pineapple salsa, fold the ends, and roll up burrito-style.

Nutrition: Calories:416; Protein:15 g; Carbs: 45 g; Sodium:545 mg; Potassium 320 mg; Fat:17 g; Calcium 130 g; Phosphorus 327 mg

BREAKFAST BAR WITH BRAN AND OATMEAL

PREPARATION: 10 min.
COOKING TIME: -
SERVING: 10 People

Ingredients:
- 1/3 cup raisins (chopped) or medium dates (diced)
- 1 cup of hot water
- 1 1/2 cups unbleached bran
- 1/2 cup flour (whole wheat)
- 1 cup of oats
- 3 tbsp sugar replacement (brown-type granular)
- a third cup of oil (corn, soybean, or safflower)

Directions:
1. Heat the water and pour it over the chopped fruit.
2. Allow for at least 15-20 minutes of standing time.
3. In a large mixing basin, combine the dry ingredients.
4. Drain the fruit and add 1 cup of hot water to the drained liquid before blending with the oil.
5. 1 minute of blending
6. Pour the liquid into the dry ingredients right away and stir well.
7. Remix in the fruit.
8. Fill a nonstick 8"x10" baking dish halfway with batter.
9. Mark cuts in 4 rows the narrow way and six rows the long way, using fingers or a spatula to level.
10. Set the oven to 380°F and bake for 20 minutes.
11. Allow cooling on a rack.
12. If you are going to store for more than two days, refrigerate or freeze.

Nutrition: Calories:149; Protein:3 g; Carbs: 20 g; Sodium:1,5 mg; Potassium 145 mg; Phosphorus 139 mg

SWEET CREPES WITH APPLES

PREPARATION: 10 min.
COOKING TIME: - min.
SERVING: 1 People

Ingredients:
- 1/2 cup unsalted butter (1 stick)
- 1 pound of flour
- 4 beaten egg yolks
- a half cup of brown sugar
- 2 eggs, whole
- Apples (three)
- 1 pound of sugar
- a quarter cup of oil
- 2 quarts of milk
- nutmeg (1/2 teaspoon)
- a half teaspoon of cinnamon

Directions:

1. Combine the egg yolks, whole eggs, sugar, flour, oil, and milk in a mixing bowl until the mixture is smooth and lump-free.
2. Over medium heat, heat a small nonstick skillet.
3. Coat the pan in cooking spray.
4. Spoon 1 scoop of batter into the pan with a 2-ounce ladle or 1/4 cup, then swirl the pan to distribute the crepe batter thinly across the bottom of the pan.
5. Cook for about 18 seconds, then turn the crepe and cook for another 10 seconds (with the help of a rubber spatula).
6. While you're making the filling, set the crepes aside.
7. Each apple should be peeled, cored, and sliced into 10-12 pieces.
8. Heat the oil in a medium sauté pan
9. Brown sugar is added to melted butter.
10. Combine the apples, cinnamon, and nutmeg in a bowl.
11. Cook and occasionally stir until the apples are tender but not mushy. Allow cooling.
12. Putting together the crepes:
13. 2 tsp apple filling in the center of each crepe
14. Create a log

Nutrition: Calories:310; Protein:6 g; Carbs: 38 g; Sodium:354 mg; Potassium 161 mg; Phosphorus 100 mg

SWEET AND CRUNCHY POPCORN

PREPARATION: 10 min.
COOKING TIME: 65 min.
SERVING: 8 People

Ingredients:

- 18 cups popcorn, popped popcorn kernels (about 3/4 cup)
- One teaspoon bicarbonate of soda
- 1 cup halved pecans
- 2 cups almonds, unblanched
- 1 pound of brown sugar
- 1 cup butter (unsalted)
- A sprinkle of cream of tartar
- 1/2 cup corn syrup

Directions:

- Layer cooked popcorn, almonds, and pecans equally in a large roasting pan.
- Combine sugar, butter, corn syrup, and cream of tartar in a big heavy pot.
- Bring to a boil over medium-high heat, continually stirring.
- Allow boiling for about 4-5 minutes, stirring occasionally.
- Remove the pan from the heat and add the baking soda.
- Pour the caramel evenly over the popcorn mixture and swirl to coat it thoroughly.
- Bake for 1 hour at about 180 degrees, stirring every 8 minutes.
- Set aside to cool, stirring once in a while.
- Keep in an airtight container for up to one week.

Nutrition: Calories:590; Protein:8 g; Carbs: 52 g; Sodium:151 mg; Potassium 255 mg; Calcium 8 g; Phosphorus 142 mg

FIBER BOOSTER BARS

PREPARATION: 10 min.
COOKING TIME: 35 min.
SERVING: 8 People

Ingredients:

- 1/5 cup applesauce
- 1 cup rolled oats
- 1/4 cup small semi-sweet chocolate chips
- 3 tbsp. chopped unsalted peanuts
- 1 tsp cinnamon powder
- 1/4 cup of crushed coconut
- Two huge eggs
- 3 tbsp honey

Directions:

1. Preheat the oven to 330 degrees Fahrenheit. Spray a 9X9-inch baking sheet with cooking spray.
2. Mix oats, cinnamon, peanuts, chocolate chips, and coconut in a large mixing bowl.
3. In a small mixing basin, whisk together the eggs. Mix in the applesauce and honey well.
4. Mix the egg mixture into the oat mixture thoroughly.
5. In a greased 9x9 pan, press the ingredients evenly into the bottom.
6. Cooking time is 35 minutes. Allow cooling before cutting into bars.
7. Keep refrigerated in an airtight container for up to one week.

Nutrition: Calories:212; Protein:7 g; Carbs: 30 g; Sodium:37 mg; Potassium 184 mg; Phosphorus 165 mg

CRANBERRY OATMEAL AND VANILLA COOKIES

PREPARATION: 10 min.
COOKING TIME: 15/20 min.
SERVING: 12 People

Ingredients:

- 1/2 cup sugar (granulated)
- A half-cup of unsalted butter
- Vanilla whey protein powder, 1.5 oz.
- A single huge egg
- One applesauce cup
- One teaspoon extract de Vanille
- A quarter cup of all-purpose flour
- salt (1/4 teaspoon)
- 3 cups oats, rolled
- 1/2 cup cranberries, dry
- A half teaspoon of cinnamon

Directions:

1. Allow butter to come to room temperature before using.
2. Preheat the oven to 350 degrees Fahrenheit. Using parchment paper, line a baking sheet.
3. Using an electric mixer, blend the butter and sugar.
4. Whisk together the egg, flour, protein powder, vanilla extract, cinnamon, and salt in a separate bowl. To blend, stir everything together.
5. Combine the applesauce with the rest of the ingredients. Combine the oats and cranberries in a mixing bowl.

6. Place 1/4 cup scoops of cookie dough on a baking pan.
7. Slightly flatten each cookie.
8. Bake for about 15 minutes, or until golden brown but still tender cookies.
9. Allow cookies to cool on the baking sheet for 5 minutes before transferring to a cooling rack to cool fully.

Nutrition: Calories:235; Protein:7 g; Carbs: 30 g; Fat: 8g; Sodium:68 mg; Potassium 123 mg; Phosphorus 98 mg

CHOCOLATE BANANA OATMEAL MORNING-BOOST

PREPARATION: 10 min.
COOKING TIME: 10 min.
SERVING: 1 Person

Ingredients:
- 1/2 cup rolled oats
- 1 cup of water
- 1/2 tiny, sliced banana
- 1 tsp of salt
- 1 tsp hazelnut-chocolate spread
- 1 tsp flaky sea salt

Directions:
- In a small saucepan, bring water and a pinch of regular salt to a boil.
- Stir in oats.
- Decrease the heat to medium, and simmer.
- Stir periodically for approximately 5 minutes or until most of the liquid has been absorbed.
- Remove the pan from the heat
- Cover, and set aside for about 3 minutes.
- Add a banana, chocolate spread, and flaky salt on the top.

Nutrition: Calories:293; Protein:7 g; Carbs: 51 g; Fat: 8g; Sodium:283 mg; Potassium 407 mg; Phosphorus 190 mg

EGG AND SAUSAGE BRUNCH

PREPARATION: 35 min.
COOKING TIME: 6 ore e 30 min.
SERVING: 15 People

Ingredients:
- 2 onion, chopped
- 1 teaspoon canola oil
- 12 slices white bread, crusts removed
- 6 ounces turkey breakfast sausage, (5 small links), casings removed
- ⅔ cup shredded extra-sharp Cheddar cheese, divided
- 1½ red bell pepper, chopped
- 1 teaspoon dry mustard
- 2½ cups low-fat milk
- ½ teaspoon salt
- ¼ teaspoon freshly ground pepper

Directions:
1. Use cooking spray to coat a 9-by-13-inch baking dish.
2. Cook sausage in a pan over medium heat until browned, crumbling with a fork.
3. Place in a mixing basin.
4. Combine the oil, onion, and bell pepper.
5. sauté and turn periodically until the veggies soften, about 6 minutes.
6. Cook and occasionally stir until the veggies brown, approximately 6 minutes longer.
7. Remove the pan from the heat and set it aside.

8. In a large mixing basin, whisk the eggs and egg whites together until well combined.
9. Combine the milk, mustard, salt, and pepper in a mixing bowl.
10. Stir 1/3 cup Cheddar cheese
11. In the baking dish, lay the bread in a thin layer.
12. Over the bread, pour the egg mixture and top with the vegetables and sausage.
13. Lastly, top with the remaining 1/3 cup of Cheddar cheese.
14. Refrigerate for at least 5/6 hours or overnight after wrapping in plastic wrap.
15. Preheat the oven to 350 degrees Fahrenheit.
16. Bake for about 50 minutes, uncovered, or until set and puffed.
17. Serve immediately.

Nutrition: Calories:147; Protein:11 g; Carbs: 13 g; Fat: 8g; Sodium:329 mg; Potassium 201 mg; Phosphorus 147 mg

STUFFED ANAHEIM CHILI PEPPERS

SERVING: 2 People

Ingredients:

- 2 Anaheim (California) green chili peppers
- 1 cup canola oil
- 3 ounces cream cheese
- 1/4 cup fresh mushrooms, sliced
- One tbs carrot
- One teaspoon onion
- One egg white
- One teaspoon all-purpose white flour

Directions:

1. Chop carrot and onion
2. Mix cream cheese, mushrooms, carrot, and onion in a mixing bowl to create the stuffing.
3. Refrigerate until you're ready to make the chili peppers.
4. Preheat a frying pan over medium-high heat
5. Place peppers in a pan and cook until the skin bubbles, flipping several times.
6. Remove the pan from the heat.
7. Peel the skin off the peppers when they're cold enough to handle.
8. Cut the chili peppers in half lengthwise and spoon half of the cream cheese stuffing inside each pepper.
9. Next, whip together the egg white and flour until stiff. Using the egg mixture, coat each stuffed chili pepper.
10. Pour enough canola oil just to cover the bottom by about one inch in a saucepan.
11. Preheat the oven to medium-high
12. Place the chili peppers in the hot oil and cook, stirring once, until golden brown. Warm it up and serve.

Nutrition: Calories:333; Protein:7.5 g; Carbs: 8.5g; Fat: 29g; Sodium:211 mg; Potassium 296 mg; Phosphorus 93 mg

PUFFED TORTILLAS BREAKFAST

PREPARATION: 35 min.
COOKING TIME: 6 ore e 30 min.
SERVING: 15 People

Ingredients:

- 2 onion, chopped
- 1 teaspoon canola oil
- 12 slices white bread, crusts removed
- 6 ounces turkey breakfast sausage, (5 small links), casings removed
- ⅔ cup shredded extra-sharp Cheddar cheese, divided
- 1½ red bell pepper, chopped
- 1 teaspoon dry mustard
- 2½ cups low-fat milk
- ½ teaspoon salt
- ¼ teaspoon freshly ground pepper

Directions:

1. Use cooking spray to coat a 9-by-13-inch baking dish.
2. Cook sausage in a pan over medium heat until browned, crumbling with a fork.
3. Place in a mixing basin.
4. Combine the oil, onion, and bell pepper.
5. sauté and turn periodically until the veggies soften, about 6 minutes.
6. Cook and occasionally stir until the veggies brown, approximately 6 minutes longer.
7. Remove the pan from the heat and set it aside.
8. In a large mixing basin, whisk the eggs and egg whites together until well combined.
9. Combine the milk, mustard, salt, and pepper in a mixing bowl.
10. Stir 1/3 cup Cheddar cheese
11. In the baking dish, lay the bread in a thin layer.
12. Over the bread, pour the egg mixture and top with the vegetables and sausage.
13. Lastly, top with the remaining 1/3 cup of Cheddar cheese.
14. Refrigerate for at least 5/6 hours or overnight after wrapping in plastic wrap.
15. Preheat the oven to 350 degrees Fahrenheit.
16. Bake for about 50 minutes, uncovered, or until set and puffed.
17. Serve immediately.

Nutrition: Calories:147; Protein:11 g; Carbs: 13 g; Fat: 8g; Sodium:329 mg; Potassium 201 mg; Phosphorus 147 mg

TASTY VEGAN BREAKFAST

PREPARATION: 15 min.
COOKING TIME: 6 min.
SERVING: 6 People

Ingredients:
- 6 oz. crumbled extra-firm or firm tofu
- 6 cups of cauliflower, or one medium head,
- Cut into tiny florets.
- 1 1/2 teaspoons of turmeric
- 2 teaspoons of avocado oil
- 1 onion, chopped and peeled
- 3 peeled and chopped garlic cloves
- 3-tablespoons with healthy yeast
- 1/2 tsp. black pepper
- Half a teaspoon of salt

Directions:
1. Put avocado oil in a pan over medium heat.
2. Once heated, add the diced onion and simmer for about 4-5 minutes until lightly caramelized and transparent.
3. Then add the garlic and stir-fry for a further 1–2 minutes until fragrant.
4. When the cauliflower is soft, add the crumbled tofu and simmer the mixture for about 5 minutes.
5. After that, season with salt, black pepper, nutritional yeast, and turmeric to taste.
6. Cook for an additional minute while stirring.
7. Distribute the mixture among six plates.

Nutrition: Calories:137; Protein:7,5 g; Carbs: 12 g; Fat: 8g; Sodium:224 mg; Potassium 408 mg.

LUNCH

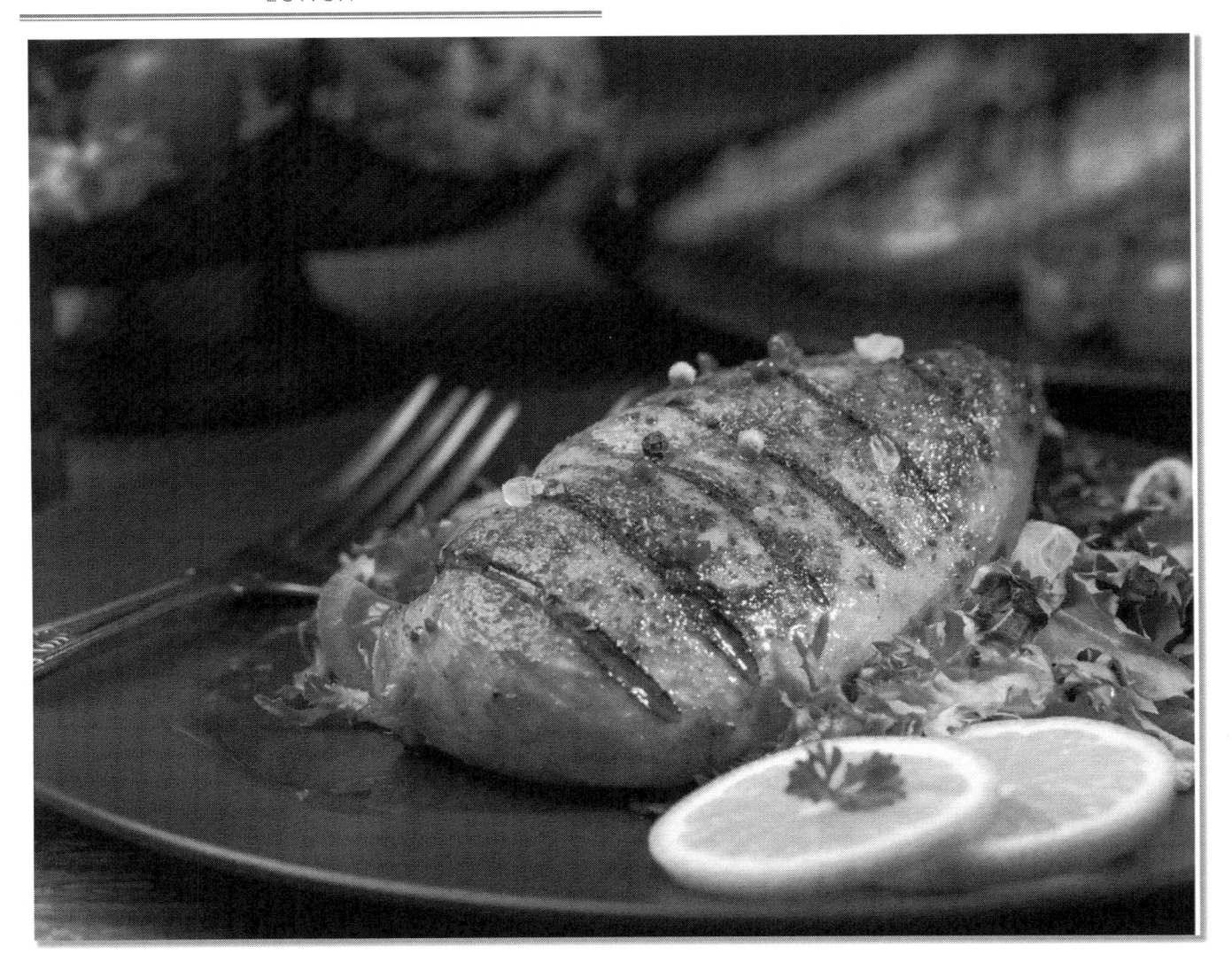

SALAD WITH VINAIGRETTE

PREPARATION: 25 min.
COOKING TIME: -
SERVING: 4 People

Ingredients:

For the vinaigrette

- Olive oil – ½ cup
- Balsamic vinegar - 4 Tbsps.
- Chopped fresh oregano – 2 Tbsps.
- Pinch red pepper flakes
- Ground black pepper

For the salad

- Shredded green leaf lettuce – 4 cups
- Carrot – 1, shredded
- Fresh green beans – ¾ cup, cut into 1-inch pieces
- Large radishes – 3, sliced thin

Directions:

1. To make the vinaigrette: put the vinaigrette ingredients in a bowl and whisk.
2. To make the salad, in a bowl, toss together the carrot, lettuce, green beans, and radishes.
3. Add the vinaigrette to the vegetables and toss to coat.
4. Arrange the salad on plates and serve.

Nutrition: Calories:273, Potassium:197mg, Phosphorous:30mg, Protein:1g, Sodium:27mg, Fat:27g

SALAD WITH LEMON DRESSING

PREPARATION: 10 min.
COOKING TIME: -
SERVING: 4 People

Ingredients:

- Heavy cream – ¼ cup
- Freshly squeezed lemon juice – ¼ cup
- Granulated sugar – 2 Tbsps.
- Chopped fresh dill – 2 Tbsps.
- Finely chopped scallion – 2 Tbsps. green part only
- Ground black pepper – ¼ tsp.
- English cucumber – 1, sliced thin
- Shredded green cabbage – 2 cups

Directions:

1. In a small bowl, stir together the lemon juice, cream, sugar, dill, scallion, and pepper until well blended.
2. Mix the cabbage and cucumber in a large bowl. Place the salad in the refrigerator and chill for 1 hour.
3. Stir before serving.

Nutrition: Calories:99, Potassium:200mg, Phosphorous:38mg, Protein:2g, Sodium:14mg, Fat:6g

SHRIMP WITH SALSA

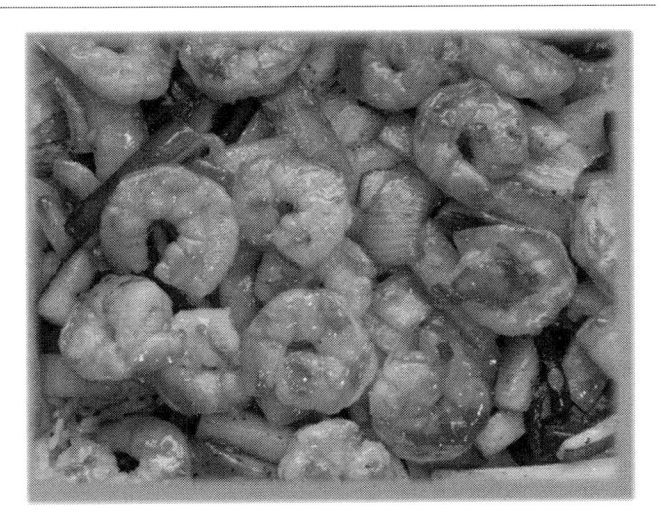

PREPARATION: 15 min.
COOKING TIME: 10 min.
SERVING: 4 People

Ingredients:

- Olive oil – 2 Tbsp.
- Large shrimp – 6 ounces, peeled and deveined, tails left on
- Minced garlic – 1 tsp.
- Chopped English cucumber – ½ cup
- Chopped mango – ½ cup
- Zest of 1 lime
- Juice of 1 lime
- Ground black pepper
- Lime wedges for garnish

Directions:

1. Soak 4 wooden skewers in water for 30 minutes.
2. Preheat the barbecue to medium heat.
3. In a bowl, toss together the olive oil, shrimp, and garlic.
4. Thread the shrimp onto the skewers, about 4 shrimp per skewer.
5. In a bowl, stir together the mango, cucumber, lime zest, and lime juice, and season the salsa lightly with pepper. Set aside.
6. Grill the shrimp for 10 minutes, turning once or until the shrimp is opaque and cooked through.
7. Season the shrimp lightly with pepper.
8. Serve the shrimp on the cucumber salsa with lime wedges on the side.

Nutrition: Calories:120, Potassium:129mg, Phosphorous:91mg, Protein:9g, Sodium:60mg, Fat:8g

CAULIFLOWER SOUP

PREPARATION: 20 min.
COOKING TIME: 30 min.
SERVING: 6 People

Ingredients:
- Unsalted butter – 1 tsp.
- Sweet onion – 1 small, chopped
- Minced garlic – 2 tsps.
- Small head cauliflower – 1, cut into small florets
- Curry powder – 2 tsps.
- Water to cover the cauliflower
- Light sour cream – ½ cup
- Chopped fresh cilantro – 3 Tbsps.

Directions:
1. In a large saucepan, heat the butter over a medium-high heat and sauté the onion-garlic for about 3 minutes or until softened.
2. Add the cauliflower, water, and curry powder.
3. Bring the soup to a boil, then reduce the heat to low and simmer for 20 minutes or until the cauliflower is tender.
4. Puree the soup until creamy and smooth with a hand mixer.
5. Transfer the soup back into a saucepan and stir in the sour cream and cilantro.
6. Heat the soup on medium heat for 5 minutes or until warmed through.

Nutrition: Calories:33, Potassium:167mg, Phosphorous: 30mg, Protein:1g, Sodium:22mg, Fat:2g

CABBAGE STEW

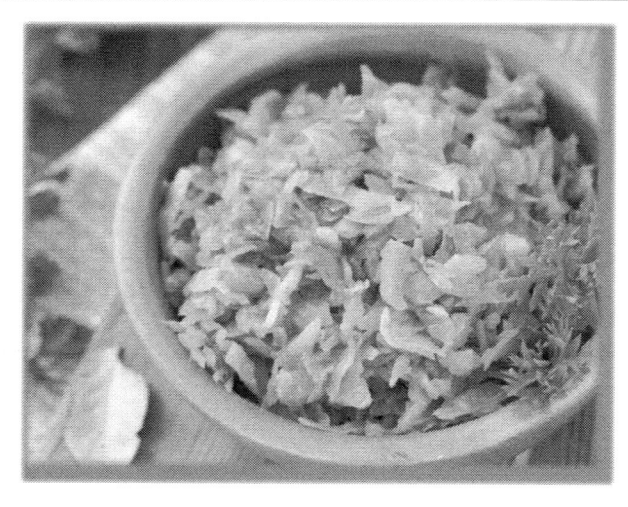

PREPARATION: 20 min.
COOKING TIME: 35 min.
SERVING: 6 People

Ingredients:
- Unsalted butter – 1 tsp.
- Large, sweet onion - ½, chopped
- Minced garlic – 1 tsp.
- Shredded green cabbage – 6 cups
- Celery stalks - 3, chopped with leafy tops
- Scallion – 1, both green and white parts, chopped
- Chopped fresh parsley – 2 Tbsps.
- Freshly squeezed lemon juice – 2 Tbsps.
- Chopped fresh thyme – 1 Tbsp.
- Chopped savory – 1 tsp.
- Chopped fresh oregano – 1 tsp.
- Water
- Fresh green beans – 1 cup, cut into 1-inch pieces
- Ground black pepper

Directions:

1. Melt the butter in a pot.
2. Sauté the onion and garlic in the melted butter for 3 minutes, or until the vegetables are softened.
3. Add the celery, cabbage, scallion, parsley, lemon juice, thyme, savory, and oregano to the pot, add enough water to cover the vegetables by 4 inches.
4. Bring the soup to a boil. Reduce the heat to low and simmer the soup for 25 minutes or until the vegetables are tender.
5. Add the green beans and simmer for 3 minutes.
6. Season with pepper.

Nutrition: Calories:33, Potassium:187mg, Phosphorous:29mg, Protein:1g, Sodium:20mg, Fat:1g

RICE AND CHICKEN SOUP

PREPARATION: 7 min.
COOKING TIME: 20 min.
SERVING: 8 People

Ingredients:

- 1 cup white onion, finely chopped
- 1 cup celery, diced
- 2 tbsp Extra virgin oil
- 1 cup baby carrot, chopped
- ½ tsp fresh ground black pepper
- ¾ cup instant white rice
- 1 bay leaf
- 4 fresh thyme sprigs
- 2 boneless skinless chicken breasts, cooked and cubed
- 10 cups no salt added chicken/vegetable broth
- 2 tbsp lime juice

Directions:

1. Sauté celery, carrot, and onion in olive oil in a large pot. Cook until softened.
2. Cook rice.
3. Add pepper, fresh thyme, bay leaf, rice, and stock. Bring to a boil.
4. Reduce heat and let simmer for 15 minutes.
5. Add chicken and cook ten minutes more.
6. Add lime juice.
7. Remove bay leaf before serving.

Nutrition: Protein -14g Carbohydrates - 19g Fat - 3g Calories - 160

HERBED CHICKEN

PREPARATION: 20 min.
COOKING TIME: 15 min.
SERVING: 4 People

Ingredients:

- Boneless, skinless chicken breast – 12 ounces, cut into 8 strips
- Egg white – 1
- Water – 2 Tbsps. divided
- Breadcrumbs – ½ cup
- Unsalted butter – ¼ cup, divided
- Juice of 1 lemon
- Zest of 1 lemon
- Fresh chopped basil – 1 Tbsp.
- Fresh chopped thyme – 1 tsp.
- Lemon slices, for garnish

Directions:

1. Place the chicken strips between 2 sheets of plastic wrap and pound each flat with a rolling pin.
2. In a bowl, whisk together the egg and 1 tbsp. water.
3. Put the breadcrumbs in another bowl.
4. Dredge the chicken strips, one at a time, in the egg, then the breadcrumbs and set the breaded strips aside on a plate.
5. In a large skillet over medium heat, melt 2 tbsps. of the butter.
6. Cook the strips in the butter for 3 minutes, turning once, or until they are golden and cooked through. Transfer the chicken to a plate.
7. Add the lemon zest, lemon juice, basil, thyme, and remaining 1 tbsp. water to the skillet and stir until the mixture simmers.
8. Remove the sauce from the heat and stir in the remaining 2 tbsps. butter.
9. Serve the chicken with the lemon sauce drizzled over the top and garnished with lemon slices.

Nutrition: Calories:255, Potassium:321mg, Phosphorous:180mg, Protein:20g, Sodium:261mg, Fat:14g

PESTO PORK CHOPS

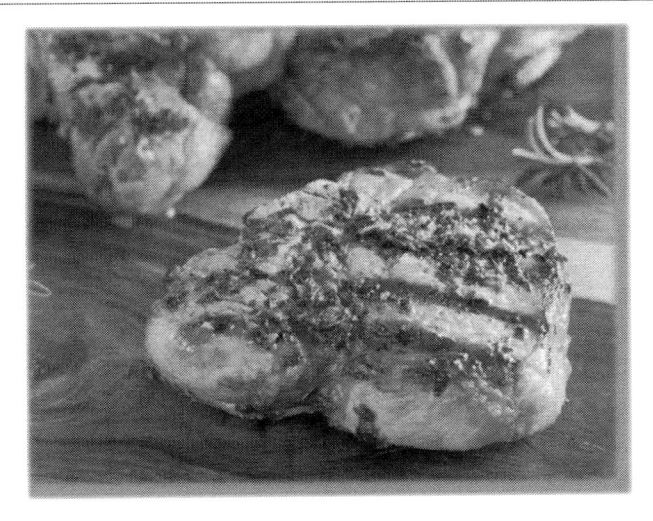

PREPARATION: 20 min.
COOKING TIME: 20 min.
SERVING: 4 People

Ingredients:

- Pork top-loin chops – 4 (3-ounce) boneless, fat trimmed
- Herb pesto – 8 tsps.
- Breadcrumbs – ½ cup
- Olive oil – 1 Tbsp.

Directions:

1. Preheat the oven to 450F.
2. Line a baking sheet with foil. Set aside.
3. Rub 1 tsp. of pesto evenly over both sides of each pork chop.
4. Lightly dredge each pork chop in the breadcrumbs.
5. Heat the oil in a skillet.
6. Brown the pork chops on each side for 5 minutes.
7. Place the pork chops on the baking sheet.
8. Bake for 10 minutes or until pork reaches 145F in the center.

Nutrition: Calories:210, Potassium:220mg, Phosphorous:179mg, Protein:24g, Sodium:148mg, Fat:7g

VEGETABLE CURRY

PREPARATION: 15 min.
COOKING TIME: 45 min.
SERVING: 4 People

Ingredients:

- Olive oil – 2 tsps.
- Sweet onion – ½, diced
- Minced garlic – 2 tsps.
- Grated fresh ginger – 2 tsps.
- Eggplant – ½, peeled and diced
- Carrot – 1, peeled and diced
- Red bell pepper – 1, diced
- Hot curry powder – 1 Tbsp.
- Ground cumin – 1 tsp.
- Coriander – ½ tsp.
- Pinch cayenne pepper
- Homemade vegetable stock – 1 ½ cups
- Cornstarch – 1 Tbsp.
- Water – ¼ cup

Directions:

1. Heat the oil in a stockpot.
2. Sauté the ginger, garlic, and onion for 3 minutes or until they are softened.
3. Add the red pepper, carrots, eggplant, and stir often for 6 minutes.
4. Stir in the cumin, curry powder, coriander, cayenne pepper, and vegetable stock.
5. Bring the curry to a boil and then lower the heat to low.
6. Simmer the curry for 30 minutes or until the vegetables are tender.
7. In a bowl, stir together the cornstarch and water.

8. Stir in the cornstarch mixture into the curry and simmer for 5 minutes or until the sauce has thickened.

Nutrition: Calories:100, Potassium:180mg, Phosphorous:28mg, Protein:1g, Sodium:218mg, Fat:3g

GRILLED STEAK WITH SALSA

PREPARATION: 20 min.
COOKING TIME: 15 min.
SERVING: 4 People

Ingredients:

Ingredients for the salsa

- Chopped English cucumber - 1 cup
- Boiled and diced red bell pepper – ¼ cup
- Scallion – 1, both green and white parts, chopped
- Chopped fresh cilantro – 2 Tbsps.
- Juice of 1 lime

For the steak

- Beef tenderloin steaks – 4 (3-ounce), room temperature
- Olive oil
- Freshly ground black pepper

Directions:

1. To make the salsa, in a bowl, combine the lime juice, cilantro, scallion, bell pepper, and cucumber. Set aside.
2. To make the steak: Preheat a barbecue to medium heat.
3. Rub the steaks all over with oil and season with pepper.
4. Grill the steaks for about 5 minutes per side for medium-rare, or until the desired doneness.
5. Serve the steaks topped with salsa.

Nutrition: Calories:130, Potassium:272mg, Phosphorous:186mg, Protein:19g, Sodium:39mg, Fat:6g

EGGPLANT AND RED PEPPER SOUP

PREPARATION: 20 min.
COOKING TIME: 40 min.
SERVING: 6 People

Ingredients:

- Sweet onion – 1 small, cut into quarters
- Small red bell peppers – 2, halved
- Cubed eggplant – 2 cups
- Garlic – 2 cloves, crushed
- Olive oil – 1 Tbsp.
- Chicken stock – 1 cup
- Water
- Chopped fresh basil – ¼ cup
- Ground black pepper

Directions:

1. Preheat the oven to 350F.
2. Put the onions, red peppers, eggplant, and garlic in a baking dish.
3. Drizzle the vegetables with the olive oil.
4. Roast the vegetables for 30 minutes or until they are slightly charred and soft.
5. Cool the vegetables slightly and remove the skin from the peppers.
6. Puree the vegetables with a hand mixer (with the chicken stock).
7. Transfer the soup to a medium pot and add enough water to reach the desired thickness.
8. Heat the soup to a simmer and add the basil.
9. Season with pepper and serve.

Nutrition: Calories:61, Potassium:198mg, Phosphorous:33mg, Protein:2g, Sodium:98mg, Fat:2g

PERSIAN CHICKEN

PREPARATION: 10 min.
COOKING TIME: 20 min.
SERVING: 5 People

Ingredients:
- Sweet onion – ½, chopped
- Lemon juice – ¼ cup
- Dried oregano – 1 Tbsp.
- Minced garlic – 1 tsp.
- Sweet paprika – 1 tsp.
- Ground cumin – ½ tsp.
- Olive oil – ½ cup
- 5 Boneless, skinless chicken thighs

Directions:
1. Put the cumin, paprika, garlic, oregano, lemon juice, and onion in a food processor and pulse to mix the ingredients.
2. Keep the motor running and add the olive oil until the mixture is smooth.
3. Place the chicken thighs in a large sealable freezer bag and pour the marinade into the bag.
4. Seal the bag and place in the refrigerator, turning the bag twice, for 2 hours.
5. Remove the thighs from the marinade and discard the extra marinade.
6. Preheat the barbecue to medium.
7. Grill the chicken for about 20 minutes, turning once, until it reaches 165F.

Nutrition: Calories:321, Potassium:220mg, Phosphorous:131mg, Protein:22g, Sodium:86mg, Fat:21g

PORK SOUVLAKI

PREPARATION: 20 min.
COOKING TIME: 12 min.
SERVING: 8 People

Ingredients:
- Olive oil – 3 Tbsps.
- Lemon juice – 2 Tbsps.
- Minced garlic – 1 tsp.
- Chopped fresh oregano – 1 Tbsp.
- Ground black pepper – ¼ tsp.
- Pork leg – 1 pound, cut in 2-inch cubes

Directions:
1. In a bowl, stir together the lemon juice, olive oil, garlic, oregano, and pepper.
2. Add the pork cubes and toss to coat.
3. Place the bowl in the refrigerator, covered, for 2 hours to marinate.
4. Thread the pork chunks onto 8 wooden skewers that have been soaked in water.
5. Preheat the barbecue to medium-high heat.
6. Grill the pork skewers for about 12 minutes, turning once, until just cooked through but still juicy.

Nutrition: Calories:95, Potassium:230mg, Phosphorous:125mg, Protein:13g, Sodium:29mg, Fat:4g

CHICKEN STEW

PREPARATION: 20 min.
COOKING TIME: 50 min.
SERVING: 6 People

Ingredients:

- Olive oil – 1 Tbsp.
- Boneless, skinless chicken thighs – 1 pound, cut into 1-inch cubes
- Sweet onion – ½, chopped
- Minced garlic – 1 Tbsp.
- Chicken stock – 2 cups
- Water – 1 cup, plus 2 Tbsps.
- Carrot – 1, sliced
- Celery – 2 stalks, sliced
- Turnip – 1, sliced thin
- Chopped fresh thyme – 1 Tbsp.
- Chopped fresh rosemary – 1 tsp.
- Cornstarch – 2 tsps.
- Ground black pepper to taste

Directions:

1. Place a large saucepan on medium heat and add the olive oil.
2. Sauté the chicken for 6 minutes or until it is lightly browned, stirring often.
3. Add the onion and garlic, and sauté for 3 minutes.
4. Add 1-cup water, chicken stock, carrot, celery, and turnip and bring the stew to a boil.
5. Reduce the heat to low and simmer for 30 minutes or until the chicken is cooked through and tender.
6. Add the thyme and rosemary and simmer for 3 minutes more.
7. In a small bowl, stir together the 2 tbsps. Of water and the cornstarch, add the mixture to the stew.
8. Stir to incorporate the cornstarch mixture and cook for about 4 minutes or until the stew thickens.
9. Remove from the heat and season with pepper.

Nutrition: Calories:141, Potassium:192mg, Phosphorous:53mg, Protein:9g, Sodium:214mg, Fat:8g

BAKED FLOUNDER

PREPARATION: 20 min.
COOKING TIME: 5 min.
SERVING: 4 People

Ingredients:

- Homemade mayonnaise – ¼ cup
- Juice of 1 lime
- Zest of 1 lime
- Chopped fresh cilantro – ½ cup
- Flounder fillets – 4 (3-ounce)
- Ground black pepper

Directions:

1. Preheat the oven to 400F.
2. In a bowl, stir together the cilantro, lime juice, lime zest, and mayonnaise.
3. Place a flounder fillet in the center of each square.
4. Top the fillets evenly with the mayonnaise mixture.
5. Season the flounder with pepper.
6. Fold the sides of the foil over the fish, creating a snug packet, and place the foil packets on a baking sheet.
7. Bake the fish for 4 to 5 minutes.
8. Unfold the packets and serve.

Nutrition: Calories:92, Potassium:137mg,

Phosphorous:208mg, Protein:12g, Sodium:267mg, Fat:4g

CARAWAY CABBAGE AND RICE

PREPARATION: 5 min.
COOKING TIME: 10 min.
SERVING: 2 People

Ingredients:

- 1 cup of rice, cooked
- ¼ cup mandarin oranges
- 1 tablespoon white onion, chopped
- 1 cup cabbage, shredded
- ½ teaspoon caraway seed
- 1 tablespoon Worcestershire sauce
- ¼ cup water

Directions:

1. Take a frying pan, grease it with oil, place it over medium heat, add onion and cabbage and cook for 4 or 5 minutes until cabbage leaves wilted.
2. Stir in caraway seeds, Worcestershire sauce, and water, continue cooking for 3 minutes, add oranges and stir until rice until well combined.
3. Serve straight away.

Nutrition: Calories:142, Potassium:194mg, Phosphorous:51mg, Protein:3g, Sodium:101 mg, Fat:0g

CHICKEN AND SWEET POTATO STIR FRY

PREPARATION: 2 min.
COOKING TIME: 40 min.
SERVING: 3 People

Ingredients:

- ¼ tsp salt
- ½ cups quinoa, rinsed and drained
- 1 clove garlic, minced
- 1 cup frozen peas
- 1 cup water
- 1 jalapeno chili pepper, chopped
- 1 medium onion, chopped
- 1 medium-sized red bell pepper, chopped
- 1 tsp cumin, ground
- 1/8 tsp black pepper
- 12oz boneless chicken
- 1med sweet potatoes, cubed
- 3 tbsp fresh cilantro, chopped
- 4 tsp canola oil

Directions:

1. Bring to a boil water and quinoa over medium heat. Simmer until the quinoa has absorbed the water.
2. In a small saucepan, put the sweet potatoes and enough water to cover the potatoes. Bring to a boil. Drain the potatoes and discard the water.
3. In a skillet, add the chicken and cook until brown. Transfer to a bowl.
4. Using the same skillet, heat 2 tablespoon of oil and sauté the onions and jalapeno pepper for one minute.

5. Add the bell pepper, cumin and garlic. Cook for three minutes until the vegetables have softened.
6. Add the peas and chicken. Cook for two minutes before adding the sweet potato and quinoa.
7. Stir cilantro and add salt and pepper to taste.
8. Serve and enjoy.

Nutrition: Calories: 415; carbs: 39g; protein: 28g; fats: 18g; phosphorus: 410mg; potassium: 1201mg; sodium: 297mg

CHICKEN AND ASPARAGUS PASTA

PREPARATION: 5 min.
COOKING TIME: 10 min.
SERVING: 8 People

Ingredients:
- 8 ounces skinless chicken breasts, cubed
- 16 ounces penne pasta, cooked
- 1 pound asparagus spears, trimmed
- ½ teaspoon minced garlic
- ¼ teaspoon garlic powder
- ½ teaspoon ground black pepper
- 1 ½ teaspoons dried oregano
- 5 tablespoons olive oil
- ¼ cup feta cheese, crumbled
- ½ cup chicken broth, low sodium

Directions:
1. Take a large skillet pan, place it over medium-high heat, add 3 tablespoons oil and when hot, add chicken cubes, stir in garlic powder and ¼ teaspoon black pepper and continue cooking for 5 minutes until cooked and browned.
2. When done, transfer chicken cubes to a plate lined with paper towels, then pour in chicken broth, add asparagus, season with oregano and remaining black pepper, and cook for 5 minutes until asparagus has steamed, covering the pan.
3. Then stir in chicken, cook for 3 minutes until warmed, stir in pasta, stir until mixed and cook for 5 minutes until hot, set aside until needed.
4. Drizzle with remaining oil, top with cheese, and serve.

Nutrition: Calories:376, Potassium:243mg, Phosphorous:193mg, Protein:18,g Sodium:110 mg, Fat:12g

HAWAIIAN RICE

PREPARATION: 5 min.
COOKING TIME: 13 min.
SERVING: 6 People

Ingredients:

- ½ cup pineapple tidbits, unsweetened
- ½ cup red bell pepper, chopped
- ½ cup mushrooms, chopped
- 1 teaspoon ginger root, minced
- ½ cup bean sprouts
- ½ tablespoon soy sauce, reduced sodium
- ¼ teaspoon salt
- 2 cups brown rice, cooked

Directions:

1. Take a frying pan, spray it with oil, place it over medium heat and when hot, add all the vegetables and cook for 5 minutes until sautéed.
2. Then stir in ginger and pineapple, drizzle with soy sauce, season with salt and cook for 3 minutes, or until hot.
3. Stir in rice until well mixed, cook for 3 minutes until hot, and then serve.

Nutrition: Calories:97, Potassium:181mg, Phosphorous:67mg, Protein:2g, Sodium:135 mg, Fat:1g

SHRIMP FRIED RICE

PREPARATION: 5 min.
COOKING TIME: 20 min.
SERVING: 4 People

Ingredients:

- 4 cups white rice, cooked
- ½ cup small frozen shrimp, cooked
- ¾ cup white onion, chopped
- 1 cup frozen peas and carrots
- 3 tablespoons scallions, chopped
- ½ teaspoon minced garlic
- 1 tablespoon ginger root, grated
- ¼ teaspoon salt
- ¾ teaspoon ground black pepper
- 5 tablespoons peanut oil
- 4 eggs

Directions:

1. Take a large skillet pan, place it over medium-high heat, add 1 tablespoon peanut oil and when hot, add onion, season with ½ teaspoon black pepper, and cook for 2 minutes, or until onions are tender.
2. Stir in scallions, ginger, and garlic, cook for 1 minute, add shrimps, stir until mixed, cook for 2 minutes until hot, then stir in carrots and peas and cook for 2 minutes until hot.
3. When done, transfer shrimps and vegetable mixture to a bowl, cover with a lid and set aside until required.
4. Return the skillet pan over medium heat, add 2 tablespoons oil, beat the eggs, pour it into the pan, cook for 3 minutes until eggs are scrambled to desired level and then transfer eggs to the bowl containing

5. shrimps and vegetables.
6. Add remaining 1 tablespoon oil and when hot, add rice, stir until well coated, and cook for 2 minutes until hot.
7. Then season rice with salt and remaining black pepper, cook for 2 minutes, don't stir, then add eggs, shrimps, and vegetables, stir until mixed and cook for 3 minutes until hot.
8. Serve straight away.

Nutrition: Calories:421, Potassium:285mg, Phosphorous: 218mg, Protein: 16g, Sodium: 271 mg, Fat:16g

VEGETARIAN EGG FRIED RICE

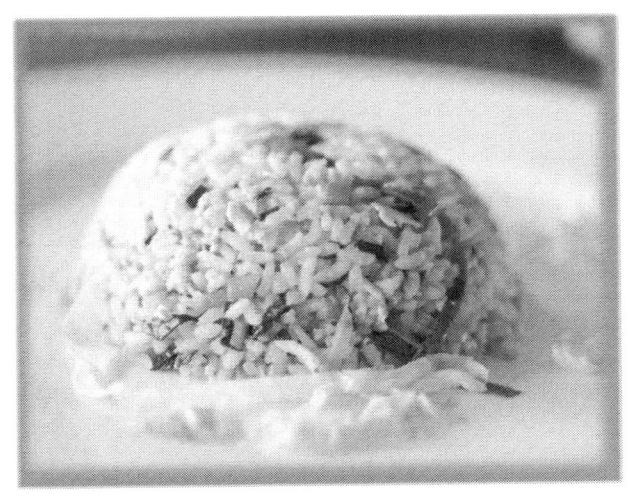

PREPARATION: 5 min.
COOKING TIME: 18 min.
SERVING: 6 People

Ingredients:
- 4 cups white rice, cooked
- 1 cup diced tofu, extra-firm, drained
- ½ cup green onion, chopped
- 1 cup white onion, diced
- 1 cup fresh carrots, sliced
- ½ cup green peas
- 1 tablespoon ginger root, grated
- 1 teaspoon minced garlic
- ¼ teaspoon mustard powder
- ½ cup cilantro, chopped
- 3 tablespoons canola oil
- 1 tablespoon soy sauce, reduced-sodium
- 6 eggs, beaten

Directions:
1. Take a large skillet pan, place it over medium heat, add oil and when hot, add beaten eggs and cook the omelet for 3 minutes until eggs are cooked to the desired level.
2. Transfer omelet to a cutting board, let it cool for 5 minutes, and chop it, set aside until needed.
3. Add oil in the pan and when hot, add all the vegetables, stir in tofu, garlic, and ginger, season with mustard, cook for 5 minutes until carrots have softened.
4. Stir in rice and chopped eggs, drizzle with soy sauce, stir until well mixed and remove the pan from heat.
5. Garnish rice with green onion and cilantro and then serve.

Nutrition: Calories: 421, Potassium: 285mg, Phosphorous: 230mg, Protein: 15g, Sodium: 238, mg, Fat: 15g

AUTUMN ORZO SALAD

PREPARATION: 35 min.
COOKING TIME: -
SERVING: 4 People

Ingredients:

- 1 medium apple, cored and diced
- ¾ cups orzo, cooked
- ¼ teaspoon ground black pepper
- 1 tablespoon fresh basil, chopped
- 2 tablespoons lemon juice
- 2 tablespoons olive oil
- 2 tablespoons almonds, sliced and blanched

Directions:

1. Take a medium-sized bowl, add all the ingredients in it (except for almonds), and stir until incorporated.
2. Take a baking dish, place prepared mixture in it, and place in the refrigerator for 30 minutes until chilled.
3. When ready to eat, garnish with almonds and serve.

Nutrition: Calories:227, Potassium: 126mg, Phosphorous:62mg, Protein:5g, Sodium:2 mg, Fat:9g

BLACKENED SHRIMP AND PINEAPPLE SALAD

PREPARATION: 10 min.
COOKING TIME: 7 min.
SERVING: 2 People

Ingredients:

- 2 cups romaine lettuce, diced
- ½ of medium red bell pepper, sliced
- 1 ½ cups pineapple chunks
- ¼ cup corn kernels
- 14 large shrimp, peeled and deveined
- 1 tablespoon blackening seasoning, low sodium
- ¼ teaspoon ground black pepper
- 1 tablespoon unsalted butter
- 1 tablespoon rice vinegar, unseasoned
- 1 tablespoon olive oil

Directions:

1. Prepare the shrimps by sprinkling them with blackening seasoning.
2. Take a skillet pan, place it over medium-high heat, add butter and when it melts, add prepared shrimps, and cook for 3 or 4 minutes per side, or until curled.
3. Transfer shrimps to a plate lined with paper towels and set aside until cooled.
4. Prepare the salad by placing all the vegetables in a large salad bowl, add corn and pineapple, season with black pepper, drizzle with vinegar and oil and toss until well mixed.
5. Top the salad with the shrimps and serve.

Nutrition: Calories:260, Potassium:468mg, Phosphorous:150mg, Protein:13g, Sodium:340mg, Fat:14g

GREEN PEPPER SLAW

PREPARATION: 5 min.
COOKING TIME: 0 min.
SERVING: 12 People

Ingredients:
- 2 medium carrots, peeled and chopped
- 1 small head of cabbage, chopped
- 1 medium green bell pepper, cored and chopped
- 2 teaspoons celery seed
- ½ cup Splenda granulated sugar
- ½ cup apple cider vinegar
- ½ cup water

Directions:
1. Take a salad bowl, place carrot, cabbage, and bell pepper in it and mix well until combined.
2. Whisk together celery seeds, sugar, vinegar, and water until blended, drizzle it over the salad and toss until mixed.
3. Serve straight away.

Nutrition: Calories:76, Potassium:108mg, Phosphorous:13mg, Protein:1g, Sodium:9mg, Fat:0g

CRANBERRIES AND COUSCOUS SALAD

PREPARATION: 10 min.
COOKING TIME: -
SERVING: 10 People

Ingredients:
- 1 cup dried cranberries, sweetened
- ½ cup green onion, chopped
- 1 ½ cups couscous, cooked
- ½ cup celery, chopped
- ½ cup cucumber, chopped
- 2 teaspoons lemon zest
- ½ teaspoon ground cumin
- 1 tablespoon parsley, chopped
- ¼ teaspoon ground cayenne pepper
- ¼ cup lemon juice
- 1 tablespoon olive oil

Directions:
1. Take a large bowl, add couscous in it, drizzle with lemon juice, season with all the spices, and stir until combined.
2. Add remaining ingredients, stir until mixed, and then serve.

Nutrition: Calories:158, Potassium:103mg, Phosphorous:55mg, Protein:4g, Sodium:11mg, Fat:2g

TUNA SALAD

PREPARATION: 10 min.
COOKING TIME: -
SERVING: 4 People

Ingredients:

- ½ of large apple, cored and chopped
- 15 ounces tuna, packed in water, unsalted
- ½ of small white onion, peeled and chopped
- 1 celery stalk, chopped
- 1/8 teaspoon salt
- 1/8 teaspoon ground black pepper
- 3 tablespoons mayonnaise
- Lettuce for serving

Directions:

1. Prepare the salad by taking a bowl, place tuna in it, add remaining ingredients in it (except for lettuce), and stir until mixed.
2. Place the salad on the lettuce and serve.

Nutrition: Calories:202, Potassium:318mg, Phosphorous:183mg, Protein:27g, Sodium:188mg, Fat:9

ROASTED VEGETABLE SALAD

PREPARATION: 10 min.
COOKING TIME: 35 min.
SERVING: 8 People

Ingredients

- 6 cups baby leaf lettuce, chopped
- 1 small head cauliflower, cut into florets
- 5 medium carrots, peeled, 2-inch diced
- ½ cup pomegranate seeds
- 1 large turnip, peeled and diced
- 1 medium white onion, peeled and diced
- ¼ teaspoon ground black pepper
- 1 tablespoon Italian seasoning blend
- ¼ teaspoon yellow mustard
- ¼ teaspoon salt
- 1 ½ tablespoons maple syrup
- 3 tablespoons rice vinegar, unseasoned
- 6 tablespoons olive oil

Directions:

1. Switch on the oven, then set it to 425ºF and let it preheat.
2. Meanwhile, take a large bowl, place all the vegetables in it, except for lettuce, season with Italian seasoning, drizzle with 3 tablespoons oil and toss until coated.
3. Take a baking sheet, place all the vegetables in it, and bake for 35 minutes until tender, turning halfway.
4. While vegetables are baking, prepare the dressing by placing remaining oil in a small bowl and whisk in salt, black pepper, mustard, vinegar, and maple syrup until combined.

5. When vegetables have roasted, transfer them to a salad bowl, add lettuce, drizzle with prepared dressing, and toss until well coated.
6. Top the salad with pomegranate seeds and then serve.

Nutrition: Calories:160, Potassium:378mg, Phosphorous:53mg, Protein:2g, Sodium:134mg, Fat:11g

CHICKEN PITA PIZZA

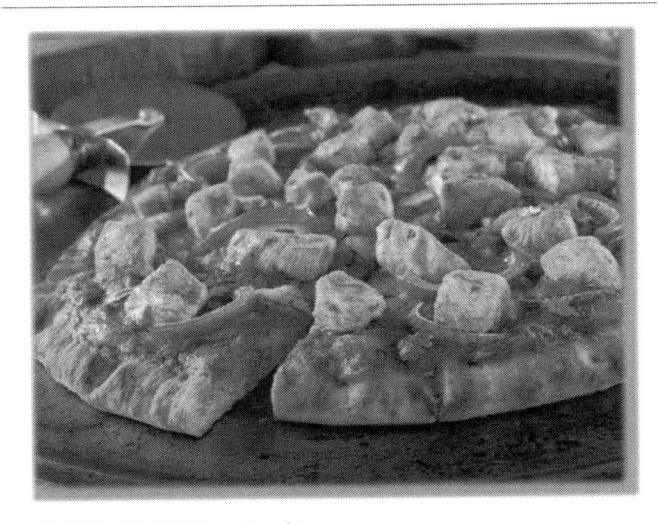

PREPARATION: 5 min.
COOKING TIME: 12 min.
SERVING: 2 People

Ingredients:
- 4 ounces chicken, cooked and cubed
- 1/8 teaspoon garlic powder
- ¼ cup purple onion, chopped
- 3 tablespoons barbecue sauce, low-sodium
- 2 tablespoons feta cheese, crumbled
- 2 pita breads, about 6 ½ inches

Directions:
1. Switch on the oven, then set it to 350ºF and let it preheat.
2. Take a baking sheet, spray it with oil, place pitas on it, spread 1 ½ tablespoon of sauce on each pita, then scatter with onions and chicken.
3. Sprinkle cheese and garlic powder on top of pitas and bake for 12 minutes until cooked.
4. Serve straight away.

Nutrition: Calories:320, Potassium:255mg, Phosphorous:221mg, Protein:23g, Sodium:523mg, Fat:9g

CHICKEN WRAPS

PREPARATION: 10 min.
COOKING TIME: 10 min.
SERVING: 4 People

Ingredients:

- 8 ounces cooked chicken, low sodium
- 1 stalk celery, diced
- ½ of medium red bell pepper, cored and diced
- ½ teaspoon onion powder
- 1 medium carrot, peeled and diced
- ¼ cup mayonnaise, low-fat
- 2 lavash, whole-wheat tortillas

Directions:

1. Place mayonnaise in a bowl, stir in onion powder until mixed and then spread 2 tablespoons of this mixture onto each bread.
2. Take a medium bowl, place all the vegetables in it, toss until mixed and distribute vegetables evenly on one side of each tortilla.
3. Roll the tortillas, then cut in half, secure with a toothpick and serve.

Nutrition: Calories:260, Potassium:215mg, Phosphorous:103mg, Protein:17g, Sodium:462mg, Fat:9g

MEXICAN CHICKEN PIZZA

PREPARATION: 10 min.
COOKING TIME: 12 min.
SERVING: 4 People

Ingredients:

- 2 cups roasted chicken breast, diced
- ½ cup red bell peppers, diced
- 1 cup kernel corn, salt-free
- ¼ cup onion, diced
- 2 tablespoons lime juice
- 4 teaspoons chopped cilantro
- ½ teaspoon minced garlic
- ½ cup shredded Monterey Jack cheese
- 4 flour tortillas, each about 6 inches

Directions:

1. Switch on the oven, then set it to 350ºF and let it preheat.
2. Then place tortillas onto a greased baking sheet and bake for 10 minutes until its edges are light brown.
3. Meanwhile, take a large skillet pan, place it over medium-high heat, grease it with oil and when hot, add corn and cook for 1 minute until corn is lightly charred.
4. Add chicken, onion, red peppers and garlic, cook for 2 minutes until hot, remove the pan from heat and then stir in lime juice until mixed.
5. When tortillas have baked, place ¾ cup of the chicken mixture on top of each tortilla, then top with 2 tablespoons of cheese and continue baking for 2 minutes, or until cheese has melted.
6. When done, sprinkle cilantro over pizza and serve.

Nutrition: Calories:309, Potassium:329mg,

Phosphorous:250mg, Protein:26g, Sodium:253mg, Fat:9g

ENERGETIC FRUITY SALAD

PREPARATION: 20 min.
COOKING TIME: 15 min.
SERVING: 12 People

Ingredients:

For Dressing:

- ½ cup of fresh pineapple juice
- 2 tbsp. of fresh lemon juice

For Salad:

- 2 cups of hulled and sliced fresh strawberries
- 2 cups of fresh blackberries
- 2 cups of fresh blueberries
- 1 cup of halved seedless red grapes
- 1 cup of halved seedless red grapes
- 6 cored and chopped fresh apples

Directions:

1. In a bowl, add all dressing ingredients and beat until well combined. Keep aside.
2. In another large bowl, mix all salad ingredients.
3. Add dressing and gently, toss to coat well.
4. Refrigerate, covered to chill before serving.

Nutrition: Per Serving: Calories: 116-Fat: 0.5g, Carbs: 29.3g, Protein: 1.2g, Fiber: 5.3g, Potassium: 276mg, Sodium: 3mg

APPEALING GREEN SALAD

COOKING TIME: 15 min.
SERVING: 4 People serving 1 salad plate

For Dressing:

- 1 tbsp. of shallot, minced
- 1/3 cup of olive oil
- 2 tbsp. of fresh lemon juice
- 1 tsp. of honey
- Freshly ground black pepper, to taste

For Salad:

- 1½ cups of chopped broccoli florets
- 1½ cups of shredded cabbage
- 4 cups of chopped lettuce

Directions:

1. In a bowl, add all dressing ingredients and beat until well combined. Keep aside.
2. In another large bowl, mix all salad ingredients.
3. Add dressing and gently, toss to coat well.
4. Serve immediately.

Nutrition: Per Serving: Calories: 179-Fat: 17.1, Carbs: 7.5g, Protein: 1.7g, Fiber: 1.9g, Potassium: 249mg, Sodium: 21mg

EXCELLENT VEGGIE SANDWICHES

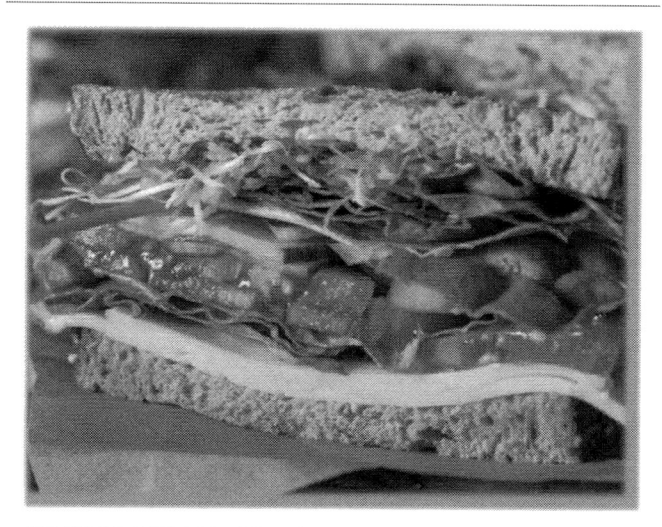

PREPARATION: 30 min.
COOKING TIME: 15 min.
SERVING: 8 People

Ingredients:

- 1 sliced large tomato
- ½ of sliced cucumber
- ½ cup of thinly sliced red onion
- 1 cup of chopped romaine lettuce leaves
- ½ cup of low-sodium mayonnaise
- 8 toasted white bread slices

Directions:

1. In a large bowl, mix together tomato, cucumber, onion and lettuce.
2. Spread mayonnaise over each slice evenly.
3. Divide tomato mixture over 4 slices evenly.
4. Cover with remaining slices.
5. With a knife, carefully cut the sandwiches diagonally and serve.

Nutrition: Per Serving: Calories: 92-Fat: 5.3g, Carbs: 10.5g, Protein: 1.2g, Fiber: 0.8g, Potassium: 112mg, Sodium: 168mg

LUNCHTIME STAPLE SANDWICHES

PREPARATION: 40 min.
COOKING TIME: 15 min.
SERVING: 2 People

Ingredients:

- 3 tsp. of low-sodium mayonnaise
- 2 toasted white bread slices
- 3 tbsp. of chopped unsalted cooked turkey
- 2 thin apple slices
- 2 tbsp. of low-fat cheddar cheese
- 1 tsp. of olive oil

Directions:

1. Spread mayonnaise over each slice evenly.
2. Place turkey over 1 slice, followed by apple slices and cheese.
3. Cover with remaining slice to make sandwich.
4. Grease a large nonstick frying pan with oil and heat on medium heat.
5. Place the sandwich in frying pan and with the back of spoon, gently, press down.
6. Cook for about 1-2 minutes.
7. Carefully, flip the whole sandwich and cook for about 1-2 minutes.
8. Transfer the sandwich into serving plate.
9. With a knife, carefully cut the sandwich diagonally ad serve.

Nutrition: Per Serving: Calories: 239-Fat: 8.5g, Carbs: 37.2g, Protein: 7g, Fiber: 5.6g, Potassium: 294mg, Sodium: 169mg

GREEK STYLE PITA ROLLS

PREPARATION: 20 min.
COOKING TIME: 15 min.
SERVING: 4 People (4 servings - serving: ½ roll)

Ingredients:
- 2 (6½-inch) pita breads
- 1 tbsp. of low-fat cream cheese
- 1 peeled, cored and thinly sliced apple
- Olive oil cooking spray, as required
- 1/8 tsp. of ground cinnamon

Directions:
1. Preheat the oven to 400 degrees F.
2. In a microwave safe plate, place tortillas and microwave for about 10 seconds to soften.
3. Spread the cream cheese over each tortilla evenly.
4. Arrange apple slices in the center of each tortilla evenly.
5. Roll tortillas to secure the filling.
6. Arrange the tortilla rolls onto a baking sheet in a single layer.
7. Spray the rolls with cooking spray evenly and sprinkle with cinnamon.
8. Bake for about 10 minutes or until top becomes golden brown.

Nutrition: Per Serving: Calories: 129, Fat: 2.2g, Carbs: 24.6g, Protein: 3.3g, Fiber: 2.1g, Potassium: 102mg, Sodium: 176mg

HEALTHIER PITA VEGGIE ROLLS

PREPARATION: 30 min.
COOKING TIME: 15 min.
SERVING: 6 People

Ingredients:
- 1 cup of shredded romaine lettuce
- 1 seeded and chopped red bell pepper
- ½ cup of chopped cucumber
- 1 small seeded and chopped tomato
- 1 small chopped red onion
- 1 finely minced garlic clove
- 1 tbsp. of olive oil
- ½ tbsp. of fresh lemon juice
- Freshly ground black pepper, to taste
- 3 (6½-inch) pita breads

Directions:
1. In a large bowl, add all ingredients except pita breads and gently toss to coat well.
2. Arrange pita breads onto serving plates.
3. Place veggie mixture in the center of each pita bread evenly. Roll the pita bread and serve.

Nutrition: Per Serving, Calories: 120-Fat: 2.8g - Carbs: 20.7g - Protein: 3.3g - Fiber: 1.5g - Potassium: 156mg - Sodium: 164mg

CRUNCHY VEGGIE WRAPS

PREPARATION: 55 min.
COOKING TIME: 15 min.
SERVING: 8 People

Ingredients:

- ¾ cup of shredded purple cabbage
- ¾ cup of shredded green cabbage
- ½ cup of peeled and julienned cucumber
- ½ cup of peeled and julienned carrot
- ¼ cup of chopped walnuts
- 2 tbsp. of olive oil
- 1 tbsp. of fresh lemon juice
- Pinch of salt
- Freshly ground black pepper, to taste
- 6 medium butter lettuce leaves

Directions:

1. In a large bowl, add all ingredients except lettuce and toss to coat well.
2. Place the lettuce leaves onto serving plates.
3. Divide the veggie mixture over each leaf evenly. Top with tofu sauce and serve.

Nutrition: Per Serving, Calories: 42-Fat: 3.1g - Carbs: 2.9g - Protein: 1.6g - Fiber: 1.1g - Potassium: 106mg - Sodium: 10mg

SURPRISINGLY TASTY CHICKEN WRAPS

PREPARATION: 50min.
COOKING TIME: 15 min.
SERVING: 4 People

Ingredients:

- 4-ounce of cut into strips unsalted cooked chicken breast
- ½ cup of hulled and thinly sliced fresh strawberries
- 1 thinly sliced English cucumber
- 1 tbsp. of chopped fresh mint leaves
- 4 large lettuce leaves

Directions:

1. In a large bowl, add all ingredients except lettuce leaves and gently toss to coat well.
2. Place the lettuce leaves onto serving plates.
3. Divide the chicken mixture over each leaf evenly.
4. Serve immediately.

Nutrition: Per Serving, Calories: 74-Fat: 2.3g - Carbs: 4.7g - Protein: 8.9g - Fiber: 0.9g - Potassium: 235mg - Sodium: 27mg

AUTHENTIC SHRIMP WRAPS

PREPARATION: 20 min.
COOKING TIME: 15 min.
SERVING: 4 People

Ingredients:

For Filling:
- 1 tbsp. of olive oil
- 1 minced garlic clove
- 1 seeded and chopped medium red bell pepper
- ½ pound of peeled, deveined and chopped medium shrimp
- Pinch of salt
- Freshly ground black pepper, to taste

For Wraps:
- 4 large lettuce leaves

Directions:
1. In a large skillet, heat oil on medium heat.
2. Add garlic and sauté for about 30 seconds.
3. Add bell pepper and cook for about 2-3 minutes.
4. Add shrimp and seasoning and cook for about 2-3 minutes.
5. Remove from heat and cool slightly. Divide shrimp mixture over lettuce leaves evenly. Serve immediately.

Nutrition: Per Serving: Calories: 97-Fat: 4.3g, Carbs: 3g, Protein: 12.6g, Fiber: 0.5g, Potassium: 81mg, Sodium: 169mg

LOVEABLE TORTILLAS

PREPARATION: 20 min.
COOKING TIME: 15 min.
SERVING: 4 People

Ingredients:
- ½ cup of low-sodium mayonnaise
- 1 finely minced small garlic clove
- 8-ounce of chopped unsalted cooked chicken
- ½ of seeded and chopped red bell pepper
- ½ of seeded and chopped green bell pepper
- 1 chopped red onion
- 4 (6-ounce) warmed corn tortillas

Directions:
1. In a bowl, mix together mayonnaise and garlic.
2. In another bowl, mix together chicken and vegetables.
3. Arrange the tortillas onto smooth surface.
4. Spread mayonnaise mixture over each tortilla evenly.
5. Place chicken mixture over ¼ of each tortilla.
6. Fold the outside edges inward and roll up like a burrito.
7. Secure each tortilla with toothpicks to secure the filling.
8. Cut each tortilla in half and serve.

Nutrition: Per Serving: Calories: 296-Fat: 8.2g, Carbs: 44g, Protein: 13.5g, Fiber: 5.9g, Potassium: 262mg, Sodium: 162mg

ELEGANT VEGGIE TORTILLAS

PREPARATION: 30 min.
COOKING TIME: 15 min.
SERVING: 12 People

Ingredients:

- 1½ cups of chopped broccoli florets
- 1½ cups of chopped cauliflower florets
- 1 tbsp. of water
- 2 tsp. of canola oil
- 1½ cups of chopped onion
- 1 minced garlic clove
- 2 tbsp. of finely chopped fresh parsley
- 1 cup of low-cholesterol liquid egg substitute
- Freshly ground black pepper, to taste
- 4 (6-ounce) warmed corn tortillas

Directions:

1. In a microwave bowl, place broccoli, cauliflower and water and microwave, covered for about 3-5 minutes.
2. Remove from microwave and drain any liquid.
3. In a skillet, heat oil on medium heat.
4. Add onion and sauté for about 4-5 minutes.
5. Add garlic and sauté for about 1 minute.
6. Stir in broccoli, cauliflower, parsley, egg substitute and black pepper.
7. Reduce the heat to medium-low and simmer for about 10 minutes.
8. Remove from heat and keep aside to cool slightly.
9. Place broccoli mixture over ¼ of each tortilla.
10. Fold the outside edges inward and roll up like a burrito.
11. Secure each tortilla with toothpicks to secure the filling.
12. Cut each tortilla in half and serve.

Nutrition: Per Serving: Calories: 217-Fat: 3.3g, Carbs: 41g, Protein: 8.1g, Fiber: 6.3g, Potassium: 289mg, Sodium: 87mg

DELIGHTFUL PIZZA

PREPARATION: 40 min.
COOKING TIME: 15 min.
SERVING: 4 People

Ingredients:

- 2 (6½-inch) pita breads
- 3 tbsp. of low-sodium tomato sauce
- 3-ounce of cubed unsalted cooked chicken
- ¼ cup of chopped onion
- 2 tbsp. of crumbled feta cheese

Directions:

1. Preheat the oven to 350 degrees F. Grease a baking sheet.
2. Arrange the pita breads onto prepared baking sheet.
3. Spread the barbecue sauce over each pita bread evenly.
4. Top with chicken and onion evenly and sprinkle with cheese.
5. Bake for about 11-13 minutes.
6. Cut each pizza in half and serve.

Nutrition: Per Serving: Calories: 133, Fat: 2g, Carbs: 18.2g, Protein: 9.8g, Fiber: 1g, Potassium: mg, Sodium: 287mg

WINNER KABOBS

PREPARATION: 50 min.
COOKING TIME: 15 min.
SERVING: 6 People

Ingredients:

- 1 pound of cubed skinless, boneless chicken breast
- 1 seeded and cut into 1-inch pieces medium red bell pepper
- 1 seeded and cut into 1-inch pieces medium green bell pepper
- 20-ounce of cut into 1-inch pieces pineapple
- 1 cut into 1-inch pieces red onion
- 1/3 cup of low-sodium barbecue sauce
- Freshly ground black pepper, to taste

Directions:

1. Preheat the outdoor grill to medium-high heat. Lightly, grease the grill grate.
2. Thread chicken, bell peppers, pineapple and onion onto pre-soaked 6 wooden skewers.
3. Coat all the ingredients with ½ of barbecue sauce and sprinkle with black pepper.
4. Place the skewers in prepared baking sheet in a single layer.
5. Grill the skewers for about 9-10 minutes, flipping occasionally.
6. Remove from grill and immediately, coat with remaining barbecue sauce. Serve immediately.

Nutrition: Per Serving: Calories: 182-Fat: 3g, Carbs: 22.2g, Protein: 18g, Fiber: 2.3g, Potassium: 234mg, Sodium: 185mg

TEMPTING BURGERS

PREPARATION: 15 min.
COOKING TIME: 10 min.
SERVING: 4 People

Ingredients:

- 12-ounce of finely chopped unsalted cooked salmon
- ½ cup of minced onion
- 1 minced garlic clove
- 2 tbsp. of chopped fresh parsley
- 1 large egg
- ½ tsp. of paprika
- Freshly ground black pepper, to taste
- 2 tbsp. of olive oil
- 3 cups torn lettuce

Directions:

1. Preheat the oven to 350 degrees F. Line a baking sheet with parchment paper.
2. In a large bowl, add all ingredients except oil and mix until well combined.
3. Make equal sized 12 patties from mixture.
4. Place patties onto prepared baking dish in a single layer.
5. Bake for about 12-15 minutes.
6. Now, in a large skillet, heat oil on high heat.

7. Remove salmon burgers from oven and transfer into skillet.
8. Cook for about 1 minute per side.
9. Divide lettuce in serving plates evenly.
10. Place 2 patties in each plate and serve.

Nutrition: Per Serving: Calories: 136, Fat: 9.1g, Carbs: 2.1g, Protein: 12.4g, Fiber: 0.5g, Potassium: 295mg, Sodium: 39mg

TASTIEST MEATBALLS

PREPARATION: 10 min.
COOKING TIME: 15 min.
SERVING: 6 People

Ingredients:
- 1 pound of lean ground chicken
- 1 tbsp. of olive oil
- 1 tsp. of minced garlic
- 2 tbsp. of minced fresh cilantro
- ½ tsp. of ground cumin
- ½ tsp. of crushed red pepper flakes
- 3 cups of torn lettuce leaves

Directions:
1. Preheat the oven to 400 degrees F.
2. Line a large baking sheet with parchment paper.
3. For meatballs in a large bowl, add all ingredients and mix until well combined.
4. Make desired sized balls from mixture.
5. Arrange the meatballs into prepared baking sheet in a single layer.
6. Bake for about 15-20 minutes or till done completely.
7. Divide lettuce in serving plates evenly. Top with meatballs and serve.

Nutrition: Per Serving: Calories: 126, Fat: 6.5 g, Carbs: 1.2g, Protein: 15.5g, Fiber: 0.5g, Potassium: 49mg, Sodium: 85mg

DINNER

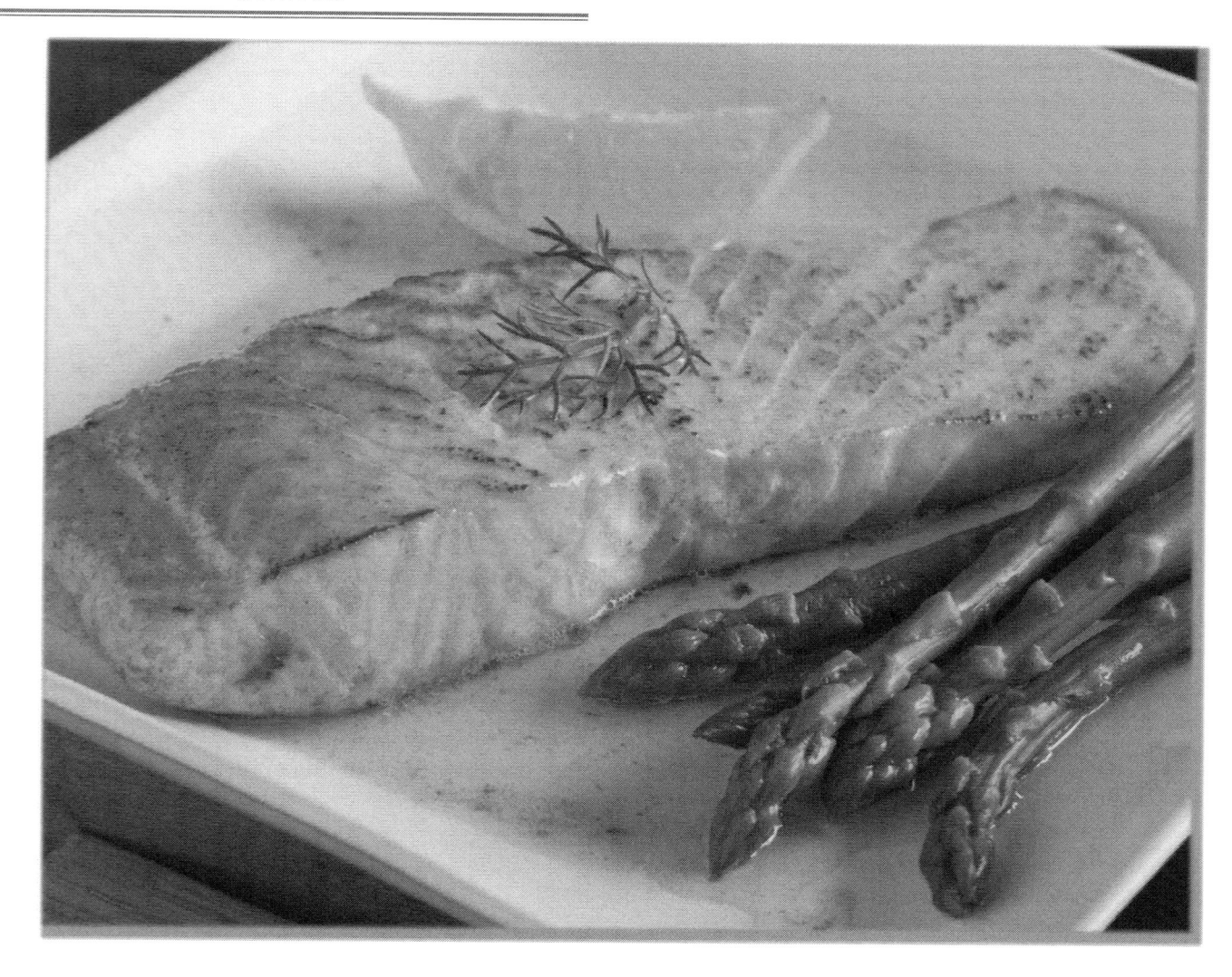

LEMON SPROUTS

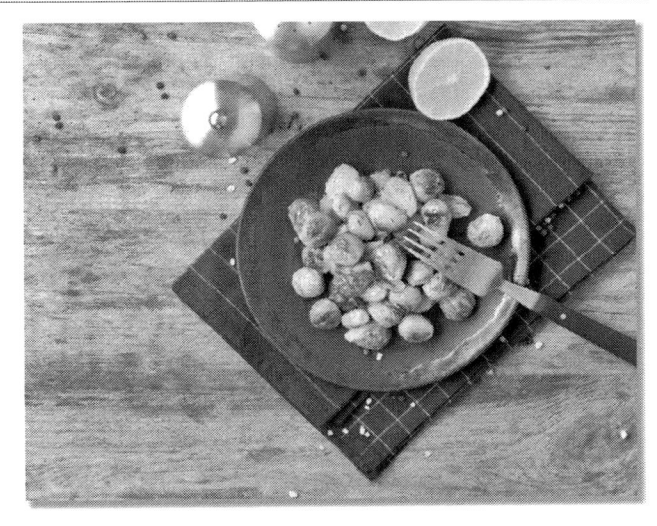

PREPARATION: 10 min.
COOKING TIME: -
SERVING: 4 People

Ingredients:
- 1 pound Brussels sprouts, trimmed and shredded
- 8 tablespoons olive oil
- 1 lemon, juiced and zested
- Salt and pepper to taste
- ¾ cup spicy almond and seed mix

Directions:
1. Take a bowl and mix in lemon juice, salt, pepper and olive oil
2. Mix well
3. Stir in shredded Brussels sprouts and toss
4. Let it sit for 10 minutes
5. Add nuts and toss
6. Serve and enjoy!

Nutrition: Calories: 382 Fat: 36g Carbohydrates: 9g Protein: 7g

LEMON AND BROCCOLI PLATTER

PREPARATION: 15 min.
COOKING TIME: 15 min.
SERVING: 6 People

Ingredients:
- 2 heads broccoli, separated into florets
- 2 teaspoons extra virgin olive oil
- 1 teaspoon salt
- ½ teaspoon black pepper
- 1 garlic clove, minced
- ½ teaspoon lemon juice

Directions:
1. Preheat your oven to 400 °F
2. Take a large-sized bowl and add broccoli florets
3. Drizzle olive oil and season with pepper, salt, and garlic
4. Spread the broccoli out in a single even layer on a baking sheet
5. Bake for 15-20 minutes until fork tender
6. Squeeze lemon juice on top
7. Serve and enjoy!

Nutrition: Calories: 49 Fat: 1.9g Carbohydrates: 7g Protein: 3g

CHICKEN LIVER STEW

PREPARATION: 10 min.
COOKING TIME: -
SERVING: 2 People

Ingredients:

- 10 ounces chicken livers
- 1-ounce onion, chopped
- 2 ounces sour cream
- 1 tablespoon olive oil
- Salt to taste

Directions:

1. Take a pan and place it over medium heat
2. Add oil and let it heat up
3. Add onions and fry until just browned
4. Add livers and season with salt
5. Cook until livers are half cooked
6. Transfer the mix to a stew pot
7. Add sour cream and cook for 22 minutes
8. Serve and enjoy!

Nutrition: Calories: 146 Fat: 9g Carbohydrates: 2g Protein: 15g

MUSHROOM CREAM SOUP

PREPARATION: 5 min.
COOKING TIME: 30 min.
SERVING: 4 People

Ingredients:

- 1 tablespoon olive oil
- ½ large onion, diced
- 20 ounces mushrooms, sliced
- 6 garlic cloves, minced
- 2 cups vegetable broth
- 1 cup coconut cream
- ¾ teaspoon salt
- ¼ teaspoon black pepper

Directions:

1. Take a large-sized pot and place it over medium heat
2. Add onion and mushrooms in olive oil and Sauté for 10-15 minutes
3. Make sure to keep stirring it from time to time until browned evenly
4. Add garlic and Sauté for 10 minutes more
5. Add vegetable broth, coconut cream, coconut milk, black pepper, and salt
6. Bring it to a boil and reduce the temperature to low
7. Simmer for 15 minutes
8. Use an immersion blender to puree the mixture
9. Enjoy!

Nutrition: Calories: 200 Fat: 17g Carbohydrates: 5g Protein: 4g

GARLIC SOUP

PREPARATION: 15 min.
COOKING TIME: 60 min.
SERVING: 10 People

Ingredients:
- 1 tablespoon olive oil
- 2 bulbs garlic, peeled
- 3 shallots, chopped
- 1 large head cauliflower, chopped
- 6 cups vegetable broth
- Salt and pepper to taste

Directions:
1. Preheat your oven to 400 °F
2. Slice ¼ inch top off the garlic bulb and place it in aluminum foil
3. Grease with olive oil and roast in the oven for 35 minutes
4. Squeeze the flesh out of the roasted garlic
5. Heat oil in a saucepan and add shallots, Sauté for 6 minutes
6. Add the garlic and remaining ingredients
7. Cover the pan and reduce the heat to low
8. Let it cook for 15-20 minutes
9. Use an immersion blender to puree the mixture
10. Season soup with salt and pepper
11. Serve and enjoy!

Nutrition: Calories: 142, Fat: 8g, Carbohydrates: 3.4g, Protein: 4g,

SIMPLE LAMB CHOPS

Preparation Time: 40 minutes
Cooking Time: 15 minutes
Serving: 2

Ingredients:
- ¼ cup olive oil
- ¼ cup mint, fresh and chopped
- 8 lamb rib chops
- 1 tablespoon garlic, minced
- 1 tablespoon rosemary, fresh and chopped

Directions:
1. Add rosemary, garlic, mint, olive oil into a bowl and mix well
2. Keep a tablespoon of the mixture on the side for later use
3. Toss lamb chops into the marinade, letting them marinate for 30 minutes
4. Place a cast-iron skillet over a medium-high heat.
5. Add lamb and cook for 2 minutes per side for medium-rare
6. Let the lamb rest for a few minutes and drizzle the remaining marinade
7. Serve and enjoy!

Nutrition: Calories: 566, Fat: 40g, Carbohydrates: 2g, Protein: 47g

GARLIC AND BUTTER-FLAVORED COD

PREPARATION: 5 min.
COOKING TIME: 20 min.
SERVING: 3 People

Ingredients:

- 3 Cod fillets, 8 ounces each
- ¾ pound baby bok choy halved
- 1/3 cup almond butter, thinly sliced
- 1 ½ tablespoons garlic, minced
- Salt and pepper to taste

Directions:

1. Preheat your oven to 400 °F
2. Cut 3 sheets of aluminum foil (large enough to fit fillet)
3. Place cod fillet on each sheet and add butter and garlic on top
4. Fold packet and enclose them in pouches
5. Arrange on baking sheet
6. Bake for 20 minutes
7. Transfer to a cooling rack and let them cool
8. Enjoy!

Nutrition: Calories: 355 Fat: 21g, Carbohydrates: 3g, Protein: 37g

TILAPIA BROCCOLI PLATTER

PREPARATION: 4 min.
COOKING TIME: 14 min.
SERVING: 2 People

Ingredients:

- 6 ounces of tilapia, frozen
- 1 tablespoon of almond butter
- 1 tablespoon of garlic, minced
- 1 teaspoon of lemon pepper seasoning
- 1 cup of broccoli florets, fresh

Directions:

1. Preheat your oven to 350 °F
2. Add fish in aluminum foil packets
3. Arrange the broccoli around fish
4. Sprinkle lemon pepper on top
5. Close the packets and seal
6. Bake for 14 minutes
7. Take a bowl and add garlic and butter, mix well and keep the mixture on the side
8. Remove the packet from the oven and transfer to a platter
9. Place butter on top of the fish and broccoli, serve and enjoy!

Nutrition: Calories: 362 Fat: 25g, Carbohydrates: 2g, Protein: 29g

PARSLEY SCALLOPS

PREPARATION: 8 min.
COOKING TIME: 23 min.
SERVING: 4 People

Ingredients:

- 8 tablespoons almond butter
- 2 garlic cloves, minced
- 16 large sea scallops
- Salt and pepper to taste
- 1 ½ tablespoons olive oil

Directions:

1. Use salt and pepper to season the scallops.
2. Take a skillet and place it over medium heat, add oil and let it heat up
3. Sauté scallops for 3 minutes per side, repeat until all scallops are cooked
4. Add butter to the skillet and let it melt
5. Stir in garlic and cook for 17 minutes
6. Return scallops to skillet and stir to coat Serve and enjoy!

Nutrition: Calories: 417, Fat: 31g, Net Carbohydrates: 5g, Protein: 29g

BLACKENED CHICKEN

PREPARATION: 10 min.
COOKING TIME: 10 min.
SERVING: 4 People

Ingredients:

- ½ teaspoon paprika
- 1/8 teaspoon salt
- 1/4 teaspoon cayenne pepper
- ¼ teaspoon ground cumin
- ¼ teaspoon dried thyme
- 1/8 teaspoon ground white pepper
- 1/8 teaspoon onion powder
- 2 chicken breasts, boneless and skinless

Directions:

1. Preheat your oven to 350 °F
2. Grease baking sheet
3. Take a cast-iron skillet and place it over high heat
4. Add oil and heat it up for 5 minutes until smoking hot
5. Take a small bowl and mix salt, paprika, cumin, white pepper, cayenne, thyme, onion powder
6. Oil the chicken breast on both sides and coat the breast with the spice mix
7. Transfer to your hot pan and cook for 1 minute per side
8. Transfer to your prepared baking sheet and bake for 5 minutes
9. Serve and enjoy!

Nutrition: Calories: 136, Fat: 3g, Carbohydrates: 1g, Protein: 24g

SPICY PAPRIKA LAMB CHOPS

PREPARATION: 10 min.
COOKING TIME: 15 min.
SERVING: 4 People

Ingredients:
- 2 lamb racks, cut into chops
- Salt and pepper to taste
- 3 tablespoons paprika
- ¾ cup cumin powder
- 1 teaspoon chili powder

Directions:
1. Take a bowl and add the paprika, cumin, chili, salt, pepper, and stir
2. Add lamb chops and rub the mixture
3. Heat grill over medium-temperature and add lamb chops, cook for 6 minutes
4. Flip and cook for 5 minutes more, flip again
5. Cook for 3 minutes, flip and cook for 2 minutes more
6. Serve and enjoy!

Nutrition: Calories: 200, Fat: 5g, Carbohydrates: 4g, Protein: 8g

STEAMED FISH

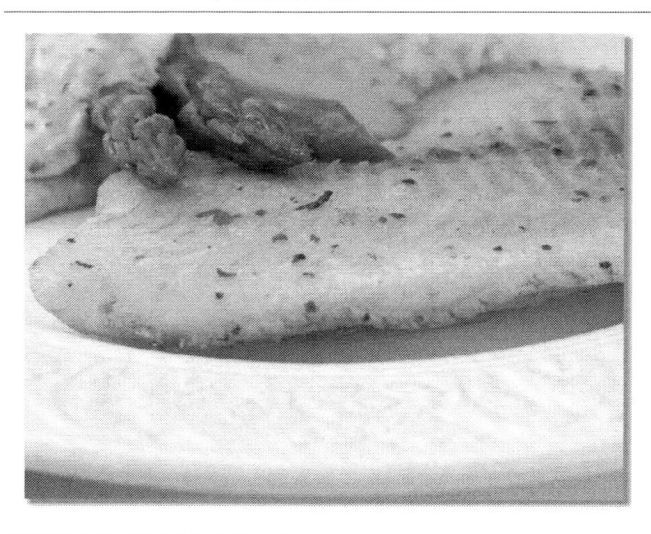

PREPARATION: 10 min.
COOKING TIME: 25 min.
SERVING: 5 People

Ingredients:
- ½ cup olive oil
- 5 fillets of tilapia
- ½ cup onion, sliced
- ¾ cup red and green peppers, sliced
- 1 tsp hot pepper sauce
- ¼ tsp black pepper
- 1 tbsp Ketchup
- 1 large sprig thyme
- 1 ½ cup hot water
- 1 tbsp lime juice

Directions:
1. In frying pan, heat the oil on medium.
2. Sauté bell peppers and onion.
3. Add ½ cup of hot water, lime juice, ketchup, thyme, hot pepper sauce, and black pepper. Stir.
4. Put fish in pan.

5. Add ½ cup of hot water. Spoon veggies and sauce over fish.
6. Cover pan and cook for 6 minutes.
7. Turn fish. Cook covered until done

Nutrition: Calories: 389, Fat: 41g, Net Carbohydrates: 10g, Protein: 29g

MUSHROOM AND OLIVE SIRLOIN STEAK

PREPARATION: 10 min.
COOKING TIME: 14 min.
SERVING: 4 People

Ingredients:
- 1-pound boneless beef sirloin steak, ¾ inch thick, cut into 4 pieces
- 1 large red onion, chopped
- 1 cup mushrooms
- 4 garlic cloves, thinly sliced
- 4 tablespoons olive oil
- 1 cup parsley leaves, finely cut

Directions:
1. Put a large skillet on the heat at a medium-high temperature
2. Add oil and let it heat up
3. Add the meat and heat it until browned on both sides. Then remove it and drain the fat.
4. Add the rest of the oil to skillet and heat it up
5. Add onions, garlic and cook for 3 minutes
6. Stir well
7. Add mushrooms olives and cook until mushrooms are thoroughly done
8. Return beef to skillet and lower heat to medium
9. Cook for 4 minutes (covered)
10. Stir in parsley
11. Serve and enjoy!

Nutrition: Calories: 386, Fat: 30g, Carbohydrates: 11g, Protein: 21g

KALE AND GARLIC PLATTER

PREPARATION: 5 min.
COOKING TIME: 10 min.
SERVING: 4 People

Ingredients:
- 1 bunch kale
- 2 tablespoons olive oil
- 4 garlic cloves, minced

Directions:
1. Carefully tear the kale into bite-sized portions, making sure to remove the stem
2. Discard the stems
3. Take a large-sized pot and place it over medium heat
4. Add olive oil and let the oil heat up
5. Add garlic and stir for 2-3 minutes
6. Add kale and cook for 5-10 minutes
7. Serve!

Nutrition: Calories: 122, Fat: 7g, Carbohydrates: 4g, Protein: 4,5g

BLISTERED BEANS AND ALMOND

PREPARATION: 10 min.
COOKING TIME: 20 min.
SERVING: 4 People

Ingredients:

- 1-pound fresh green beans, ends trimmed
- 1 ½ tablespoon olive oil
- ¼ teaspoon salt
- 1 ½ tablespoons fresh dill, minced
- Juice of 1 lemon
- ¼ cup crushed almonds
- Salt as needed

Directions:

1. Preheat your oven to 400 °F
2. Add in the green beans with your olive oil and the salt
3. Then spread them in one single layer on a large-sized sheet pan
4. Roast for 12 minutes and stir nicely, then roast for another 9-10 minutes
5. Remove it from the oven and keep stirring in the lemon juice alongside the dill
6. Top it with crushed almonds, some flaky sea salt and serve

Nutrition: Calories: 347, Fat: 16g, Carbohydrates: 6g, Protein: 45g

EGGPLANT CRUNCHY FRIES

PREPARATION: 10 min.
COOKING TIME: 10 min.
SERVING: 6 People

Ingredients:

- 1 eggplant – medium size
- 2 eggs
- 5 tablespoons cornstarch
- 5 tablespoons breadcrumbs
- 1 teaspoon garlic powder
- ½ cup oil – canola or olive oil

Direction:

1. Clean and peel the eggplant and cut it in French fries-like sticks. Make sure that you dry the sticks not to be too moisty.
2. In the meanwhile, beat the eggs until foamy and combine cornstarch, garlic powder and breadcrumbs in another bowl.
3. Heat the oil in a skillet.
4. Once the oil is hot, start dipping eggplant dip into the egg mixture, then coat the sticks with the cornstarch and breadcrumbs mixture.
5. Fry the coated sticks for around 3 minutes, flipping them over to brown them on all sides
6. Serve hot.

Nutrition: Potassium 215 mg, Sodium 212 mg, Phosphorus 86 mg, Calories 233

OREGANO SALMON WITH CRUNCHY CRUST

PREPARATION: 10 min.
COOKING TIME: 2 hours
SERVING: 2 People

Ingredients:
- 8 oz salmon fillet
- 2 tablespoons panko breadcrumbs
- 1 oz Parmesan, grated
- 1 teaspoon dried oregano
- 1 teaspoon sunflower oil

Directions:
1. In the mixing bowl combine together panko breadcrumbs, Parmesan, and dried oregano.
2. Sprinkle the salmon with olive oil and coat in the breadcrumb's mixture.
3. After this, line the baking tray with baking paper.
4. Place the salmon in the tray and transfer in the preheated to the 385F oven.
5. Bake the salmon for 25 minutes.

Nutrition: calories 245, fat 12.8, fiber 0.6, carbs 5.9, protein 27.5

BROILED SHRIMP

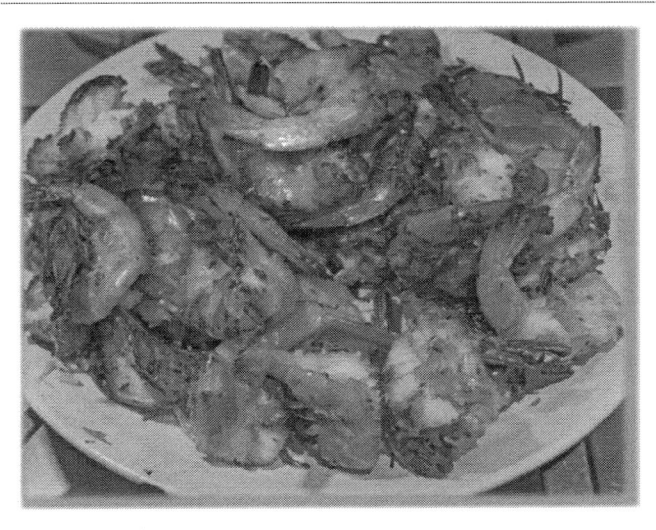

PREPARATION: -
COOKING TIME: 5 min.
SERVING: 8 People

Ingredients:
- 1 lb. shrimp in shell
- 1/2 cup unsalted butter, melted
- 2 teaspoons lemon juice
- 2 tablespoons chopped onion
- 1 clove garlic, minced
- 1/8 teaspoon pepper

Directions:
1. Toss the shrimp with the butter, lemon juice, onion, garlic, and pepper in a bowl.
2. Spread the seasoned shrimp in a baking tray.
3. Broil for 5 minutes in an oven on broiler setting.
4. Serve warm.

Nutrition: calories 167, fat 12.8, fiber 0.1, carbs 0.6, protein 14.6

SHRIMP SPAGHETTI

PREPARATION: 10 min.
COOKING TIME: 40 min.
SERVING: 4 People

Ingredients:
- 1/3 cup extra virgin olive oil
- ½ lb. spaghetti or spaghettini
- 2 cloves garlic, crushed
- 1/3 cup dry white wine
- 1 red pepper, diced
- 1/4 tsp crushed red chilies
- 1/3 cup toasted fresh breadcrumbs
- 1 lb. raw shrimp
- Chopped fresh parsley (optional)
- Freshly ground pepper, to taste

Directions:
1. Cook pasta.
2. Heat the oil in a large skillet over medium-low.
3. Add crushed the red chilies and garlic. Cook, stirring, for 1 minute.
4. Add peppers, cooking for 5 minutes.
5. Add the shrimp. Cook for 1 minute.
6. Add the wine.
7. Turn the heat up to medium. Simmer until the shrimp start to curl and turn opaque.
8. Drain pasta. Put it in a large serving dish.
9. Pour sauce over pasta. Toss together with breadcrumbs.
10. Serve with parsley and freshly ground pepper.

Nutrition: calories 716, fat 55, fiber 0, carbs 25, protein 25

TERIYAKI TUNA

PREPARATION: 10 min.
COOKING TIME: 6 min.
SERVING: 3 People

Ingredients:
- 3 tuna fillets
- 3 teaspoons teriyaki sauce
- ½ teaspoon minced garlic
- 1 teaspoon olive oil

Directions:
1. Whisk together teriyaki sauce, minced garlic, and olive oil.
2. Brush every tuna fillet with teriyaki mixture.
3. Preheat grill to 390F.
4. Grill the fish for 3 minutes from each side.

Nutrition: calories 382, fat 32.6, fiber 0, carbs 1.1, protein 21.4

CHICKEN NOODLE SOUP

PREPARATION: 15 min.
COOKING TIME: 25 min.
SERVING: 4 People

Ingredients:
- 1 cup low-sodium chicken broth
- 1 cup water
- 1/4 teaspoon poultry seasoning
- 1/4 teaspoon black pepper
- 1/4 cup carrot, chopped
- 1 cup chicken, cooked and shredded
- 2 ounces egg noodles

Direction:
1. Add broth and water in a slow cooker.
2. Set the pot to high.
3. Add poultry seasoning and pepper.
4. Add carrot, chicken, and egg noodles to the pot.
5. Cook on high setting for 25 minutes.
6. Serve while warm.

Nutrition: Calories 141, Protein 15 g, Carbohydrates 11 g, Fat 4 g, Cholesterol 49 mg, Sodium 191 mg, Potassium 135 mg, Phosphorus 104 mg, Calcium 16 mg, Fiber 0.7 g

BEEF STEW WITH APPLE CIDER

PREPARATION: 15 min.
COOKING TIME: 10 min.
SERVING: 8 People

Ingredients:
- 1/2 cup potatoes, cubed
- 2 lb. beef cubes
- 7 tablespoons all-purpose flour, divided
- 1/4 teaspoon thyme
- Black pepper to taste
- 3 tablespoons oil
- ¼ cup carrot, sliced
- 1 cup onion, diced
- 1/2 cup celery, diced
- 1 cup apples, diced
- 2 cups apple cider
- 1/2 cups water
- 2 tablespoons apple cider vinegar

Direction:
1. Double boil the potatoes (to reduce the amount of potassium) in a pot of water.
2. In a shallow dish, mix the half of the flour, thyme and pepper.
3. Coat all sides of beef cubes with the mixture.
4. In a pan over medium heat, add the oil and cook the beef cubes until brown. Set aside.
5. Layer the ingredients in your slow cooker.
6. Put the carrots, potatoes, onions, celery, beef and apple.
7. In a bowl, mix the cider, vinegar and 1 cup water.
8. Add this to the slow cooker.
9. Cook on low setting for 10 hours.
10. Stir in the remaining flour to thicken the soup.

Nutrition: Calories 365, Protein 33 g, Carbohydrates 20g, Fat 17g, Cholesterol 73 mg,

Sodium 80 mg, Potassium 540 mg, Phosphorus 234 mg, Calcium 36 mg, Fiber 2.2 g

CHICKEN CHILI

PREPARATION: 20 min.
COOKING TIME: 1 hour and 15 min.
SERVING: 8 People

Ingredients:

- 1 tablespoon oil
- 1 cup onion, chopped
- 4 garlic cloves, chopped
- 1 cup green pepper
- 1 cup celery, chopped
- 1 cup carrots, chopped
- 14 oz. low-sodium chicken broth
- 1 lb. chicken breast, cubed and cooked
- 1 cup low-sodium tomatoes, drained and iced
- 1 cup kidney beans, rinsed and drained
- 3/4 cup salsa
- 3 tablespoons chili powder
- 1 teaspoon ground oregano
- 4 cups white rice, cooked

Direction:

1. In a pot, pour oil and cook onion, garlic, green pepper, celery, and carrots.
2. Add the broth.
3. Bring to a boil.
4. Add the rest of the ingredients except the rice.
5. Simmer for 1 hour.
6. Serve with rice.

Nutrition: Calories 355, Protein 24 g, Carbohydrates 38 g, Fat 12 g, Cholesterol 59 mg, Sodium 348 mg, Potassium 653 mg, Phosphorus 270 mg, Calcium 133 mg, Fiber 4.7g

TOFU STIR FRY

PREPARATION: 15 min.
COOKING TIME: 20 min.
SERVING: 4 People

Ingredients:

- 1 teaspoon sugar
- 1 tablespoon lime juice
- 1 tablespoon low sodium soy sauce
- 2 tablespoons cornstarch
- 2 egg whites, beaten
- 1/2 cup unseasoned breadcrumbs
- 1 tablespoon vegetable oil
- 16 ounces tofu, cubed
- 1 clove garlic, minced
- 1 tablespoon sesame oil
- 1 red bell pepper, sliced into strips
- 1 cup broccoli florets
- 1 teaspoon herb seasoning blend
- Dash black pepper
- Sesame seeds
- Steamed white rice

Direction:

1. Dissolve sugar in a mixture of lime juice and soy sauce. Set aside.
2. In the first bowl, put the cornstarch.
3. Add the egg whites in the second bowl.
4. Place the breadcrumbs in the third bowl.
5. Dip each tofu cubes in the first, second and third bowls.
6. Pour vegetable oil in a pan over medium heat.
7. Cook tofu cubes until golden.
8. Drain the tofu and set aside.
9. Remove oil from the pan and add sesame oil.
10. Add garlic, bell pepper and broccoli.
11. Cook until crisp tender.

12. Season with the seasoning blend and pepper.
13. Put the tofu back and toss to mix.
14. Pour soy sauce mixture on top and transfer to serving bowls.
15. Garnish with the sesame seeds and serve on top of white rice.

Nutrition: Calories 400, Protein 19 g, Carbohydrates 45g, Fat 16g, Cholesterol 0 mg, Sodium 584 mg, Potassium 317 mg, Phosphorus 177 mg, Calcium 253 mg, Fiber 2.7 g

BROCCOLI PANCAKE

PREPARATION: 10 min.
COOKING TIME: 5 min.
SERVING: 4 People

Ingredients:

- 3 cups broccoli florets, diced
- 2 eggs, beaten
- 2 tablespoons all-purpose flour
- ½ cup onion, chopped
- 2 tablespoons olive oil

Direction:

1. Boil broccoli in water for 5 minutes. Drain and set aside.
2. Mix egg and flour.
3. Add onion and broccoli to the mixture.
4. Pour oil in a pan over medium heat.
5. Cook the broccoli pancake until brown on both sides.

Nutrition: Calories 140, Protein 6 g, Carbohydrates 7 g, Fat 10 g, Cholesterol 106 mg, Sodium 58 mg, Potassium 276 mg, Phosphorus 101 mg, Calcium 50 mg, Fiber 2.1 g

TANGY WHOLE ROASTED SEA BASS WITH OREGANO

PREPARATION: 15 min.
COOKING TIME: 20 min.
SERVING: 4 People

Ingredients

- 2 medium-sized whole sea bass
- 1 tbsp. extra virgin olive oil
- 2 garlic cloves, thinly sliced
- ½ tsp. dried oregano
- 2 tsp. freshly squeezed lemon juice
- Kosher salt and freshly ground pepper, to taste
- 2 lemons, thinly sliced

Directions:

1. Start by preheating your broiler or grill to medium-high heat. Lightly grease the rack with olive oil cooking spray.

2. Combine the lemon juice, olive oil, salt, pepper and oregano in a bowl and let stand. Use a sharp knife to make 3 horizontal slits on each side of the fish and rub with some kosher salt. Use a brush to rub in the lemon-herb mixture in the slits.

3. Cook the fish in the reheated broiler/grill for about 15-20 minutes, turning twice in between cook time and baste with the lemon-oregano mixture. Grill until the flesh turns opaque or until desired doneness is achieved.

4. Let the sea bass rest for 50-10 minutes before serving. Serve with steamed veggies or a salad.

5. Enjoy!

Nutrition: Calories: 236; Total Fat: 16g; Carbs: 2g; Dietary Fiber 1g; Protein: 37g; Cholesterol: 0mg; Sodium: 563mg

PAN-SEARED SALMON SALAD WITH LEMON-DRESSING

PREPARATION: 15 min.
COOKING TIME: -
SERVING: 4 People

Ingredients

- 4 (100g) skin-on salmon fillets
- 1/8 teaspoon sea salt
- 2 teaspoons extra virgin olive oil
- 4 cups arugula
- 8 leaves Boston lettuce, washed and dried
- 1 cup snow peas, cooked

For Lemon-Dill Dressing:

- 1/4 cup lemon juice
- 1/4 cup extra virgin olive oil
- 1 teaspoon raw honey
- 1 tablespoon Dijon mustard
- 1 tablespoon chopped fresh dill
- 2 garlic cloves, minced
- 1/2 teaspoon salt

Directions:

1. Sprinkle fish with about 1/8 teaspoon salt and cook in 2 teaspoons of olive oil over medium heat for about 4 minutes per side or until golden.

2. In a small bowl, whisk together al dressing ingredients and set aside.

3. Divide arugula and lettuce among four serving plates

4. Divide lettuce and arugula among 4 plates and add the remaining salad ingredients, top each with seared salmon and drizzle with dressing. Enjoy!

Nutrition: Calories: 608; Total Fat: 46 g; Carbs: 16.2 g; Dietary Fiber: 8.7 g; Sugars: 5.1 g; Protein: 38.9 g; Cholesterol: 78 mg; Sodium: 488 mg

GRILLED STEAK SERVED WITH CREAMY PEANUT SAUCE

PREPARATION: 10 min.
COOKING TIME: 10 min.
SERVING: 4 People

Ingredients:

For the salads

- 3 pounds steak, sliced
- 4 tablespoons olive oil
- ½ cup chopped red onion
- 4 cloves garlic, minced
- Salt and pepper

Sauce

- 1 cup coconut cream
- 4 tablespoons natural peanut butter
- 8-10 chives
- 1 clove of garlic, chopped
- 4 fresh basil leaves
- 1 teaspoon dried minced red onion
- A sprig fresh rosemary
- 1/2 teaspoon dried dill
- A few leaves of fresh parsley
- 1/2 liquid stevia
- pinch of chicory powder
- 1/4 teaspoon sea salt
- Pinch of pepper

Directions:

1. Heat olive oil in a skillet until hot but not smoky; add onion and garlic; sauté until tender. Add in steak pieces and fry until browned and cooked through. Season with salt and pepper and set aside.
2. In a food processor or blend, blend together dressing ingredients until very smooth.
3. Serve steak drizzled with the sauce.

Nutrition: Calories: 480; Total Fat: 28.1 g; Carbs: 9.3 g; Dietary fiber: 2.5 g; Sugars: 4.6 g; Protein: 49 g; Cholesterol: 131 mg; Sodium: 854 mg

LEAN STEAK WITH OREGANO-LEMON CHIMICHURRI & ARUGULA SALAD

PREPARATION: 5 min.
COOKING TIME: 5 min.
SERVING: 4 People

Ingredients:

- 1 teaspoon finely grated lemon zest
- 1 teaspoon dried oregano
- 1 small garlic clove, grated
- 2 teaspoon apple cider vinegar
- 1 tablespoon fresh lemon juice
- 1/2 cup chopped fresh flat-leaf parsley leaves
- 1 1/2-pound lean steak, cut into 4 pieces
- Sea salt and pepper
- 1/4 cup and 2 teaspoons extra virgin olive oil
- 4 cups arugula
- 2 bulbs fennel, shaved
- 2 tablespoons mustard

Directions:

1. Make chimichurri: In a medium bowl, combine lemon zest, oregano, and garlic. Mix in vinegar, lemon juice and parsley and then slowly whisk in ¼ cup of olive oil until emulsified. Season with sea salt and pepper.
2. Sprinkle the steak with salt and pepper; heat the remaining olive oil in a large skillet and cook steak over medium high heat for about 6 minutes per side or until browned. Remove from heat and let rest for at least 10 minutes.
3. Toss steak, greens, and fennel with mustard in a medium bowl, season with salt and pepper.
4. Serve steak with chimichurri and salad. Enjoy!

Nutrition: Calories: 343; Total Fat: 20.6 g; Carbs: 2 g; Dietary Fiber: 0.5 g; Sugars: 0.8 g; Protein: 0.6 g; Cholesterol: 99 mg; Sodium: 146 mg

HERBED LONDON BROIL

PREPARATION: 10 min.
COOKING TIME: 30 min.
SERVING: 1 Person

Ingredients:

- 100 grams lean London broil,
- sliced thinly into strips
- 1 clove garlic, minced
- 1 red onion, minced
- ¼ cup beef broth or water
- Chopped Italian parsley
- Pinch of rosemary
- 1/8 teaspoon thyme
- Pinch of salt & pepper

Directions:

1. Coat beef with salt and pepper and add to a pan along with beef broth and herbs; cook until beef is cooked through. Serve garnished with parsley.

Nutrition: Calories: 201; Total Fat: 6.6 g; Carbs: 1.4 g; Dietary Fiber: 0.4 g; Sugars: 0.6 g; Protein: 31.7 g; Cholesterol: 89 mg; Sodium: 257 mg

GROUND BEEF TACOS

PREPARATION: 10 min.
COOKING TIME: 25 min.
SERVING: 1 Person

Ingredients:

- 100 grams lean ground beef
- 1 clove garlic, minced
- ½ red onion, minced
- Lettuce leaves
- Cayenne pepper
- Fresh chopped cilantro
- Pinch of dried oregano
- Dash of onion powder
- Dash of garlic powder
- Pinch of salt & pepper

Directions:

1. Fry beef in a splash of lemon juice until browned; add garlic, onion and spices, and water and simmer for about 5-10 minutes. Season with salt and serve taco style in romaine lettuce or butter lettuce or with a side of salsa or tomatoes.

Nutrition: Calories: 194; Total Fat: 6.3 g; Carbs: 1.9 g; Dietary Fiber: 0.5 g; Sugars: 0.7 g; Protein: 30.6 g; Cholesterol: 89 mg; Sodium: 67 mg

PEPPER CRUSTED STEAK

PREPARATION: 10 min.
COOKING TIME: 5 min.
SERVING: 1 Person

Ingredients

- 100 grams lean steak
- Dash of Worcestershire sauce
- Pinch of salt & pepper

Directions:

1. Pound meat until tender and flat; rub with salt and pepper and cook on high heat for about 3-5 minutes. Serve topped with Worcestershire sauce and garnished with caramelized onions.

Nutrition: Calories: 189; Total Fat: 6.2 g; Carbs: 0.2 g; Dietary Fiber: 0 g; Sugars: 0.1 g; Protein: 30.4 g; Cholesterol: 89 mg; Sodium: 228 mg

STIR-FRIED CHICKEN WITH WATER CHESTNUTS

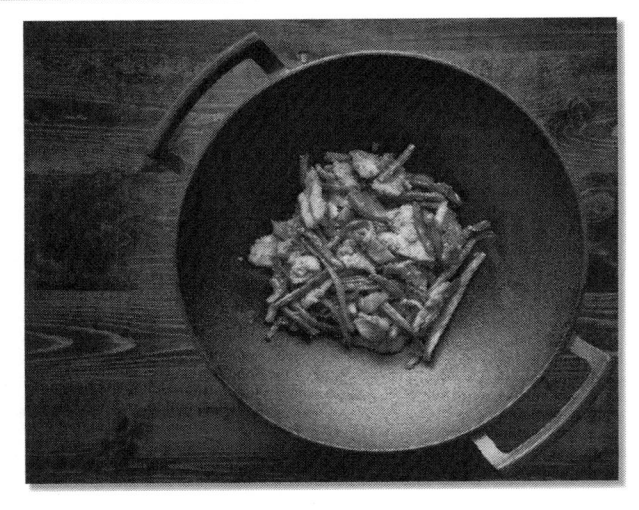

PREPARATION: 10 min.
COOKING TIME: 15 min.
SERVING: 4 People

Ingredients:

- 2 tablespoons sesame oil
- ¼ cup wheat-free tamari
- 4 small chicken breasts, sliced
- 1 small cabbage, chopped
- 3 garlic cloves, chopped
- ¼ teaspoons peppercorns
- ¼ teaspoon ground fennel seeds
- 1/4 teaspoon cinnamon
- 1/4 teaspoon ground cloves
- ¼ teaspoon star anise
- 1 cup dried plums
- 1 cup water chestnuts
- Toasted sesame seeds

Directions:

1. Heat sesame oil in a large skillet set over medium heat; stir in all the ingredients, except sesame seeds, and cook until cabbage and chicken are tender.
2. Serve warm sprinkled with toasted sesame seeds.

Nutrition: Calories: 306; Total Fat: 13.5 g; Carbs: 23.4 g; Dietary Fiber: 0.7 g; Sugars: 2 g; Protein: 22.5 g; Cholesterol: 62 mg; Sodium: 29 mg

LEMON GARLIC SALMON

PREPARATION: 15 min.
COOKING TIME: 30 min.
SERVING: 4 People

Ingredients:

- 1 teaspoon extra virgin olive oil
- 4 salmon fillets
- 3 tablespoons freshly squeezed lemon juice
- 1 tablespoon coconut milk
- 1 teaspoon ground pepper
- 1 teaspoon dried parsley flakes
- 1 finely chopped clove garlic

Directions:

1. Preheat your oven to 190°C (275°F). Coat a baking dish with extra virgin olive oil.
2. Rinse the fish under water and pat dry with paper towels.
3. Arrange the fish fillet in the coated baking dish and drizzle with lemon juice and coconut oil. Sprinkle with ground pepper, parsley and garlic.
4. Bake in the oven for about 30 minutes or until it flakes easily when touched with a fork.

Nutrition: Calories: 248; Total Fat: 12g; Carbs: 0.7g; Dietary Fiber: trace; Protein: 34.8g; Cholesterol: 0mg; Sodium: 82mg; trace

PAN-FRIED CHILI BEEF WITH TOASTED CASHEWS

PREPARATION: 10 min.
COOKING TIME: 25 min.
SERVING: 4 People

Ingredients:

- ½ tablespoon extra-virgin olive oil or canola oil
- 1-pound sliced lean beef
- 2 teaspoons red curry paste
- 1 teaspoon raw honey
- 2 tablespoons fresh lime juice
- 2 teaspoon fish sauce
- 1 cup green capsicum, diced
- ½ cup water
- 24 toasted cashews
- 1 teaspoon arrowroot

Directions:

1. Add oil to a pan set over medium heat; add beef and fry until it's no longer pink inside. Stir in red curry paste and cook for a few more minutes.
2. Stir in honey, lime juice, fish sauce, capsicum and water; simmer for about 10 minutes.
3. Mix cooked arrowroot with water to make a paste; stir the paste into the sauce to thicken it. Remove the pan from heat and add the fried cashews. Serve.

Nutrition: Calories: 361; Total Fat: 17.7 g; Carbs: 12.9 g; Dietary Fiber: 1.2 g; Sugars: 3.8 g; Protein: 38 g; Cholesterol: 101 mg; Sodium: 444 mg

HEALTHY KETO COCONUT-LIME SKIRT STEAK

PREPARATION: 10 min.
COOKING TIME: 30 min.
SERVING: 4 People

Ingredients:

- 2 pounds skirt steak, cut into sections
- 2 tbsp. fresh lime juice
- 1/2 cup melted coconut oil
- 1 tsp red pepper flakes
- 1 tsp grated fresh ginger
- 1 tbsp. minced garlic
- zest of one lime
- 3/4 tsp sea salt

Directions:

1. In a bowl, mix together lime juice, coconut oil, red pepper flakes, ginger, garlic, lime zest and salt until well combined.

2. Toss in steak and marinate for at least 20 minutes; transfer the meat to a skillet set over medium heat and spoon over the marinade.

3. Sear the meat for about 5 minutes per side or until cooked through and golden brown.

4. Serve and enjoy!

Nutrition: Calories: 661; Total Fat: 54g; Carbs: 5g; Dietary Fiber: 0g; Sugars: 1g; Protein: 35g.

SPICY GRILLED COD

PREPARATION: 15 min.
COOKING TIME: 20 min.
SERVING: 4 People

Ingredients:
- 1-pound cod filets
- 2 tablespoons extra-virgin olive oil
- 2 minced garlic cloves
- 1/8 teaspoon cayenne pepper
- 3 tablespoons fresh lime juice
- 1 ½ teaspoon fresh lemon juice
- ¼ cup freshly squeezed orange juice
- 1/3 cup water
- 2 tablespoon chopped fresh chives

Direction:
1. In a bowl, mix together lemon, lime juice, orange, cayenne pepper, extra virgin olive oil, garlic and water.
2. Place fish in a dish and add the marinade, reserving ¼ cup; marinate in the refrigerator for at least 30 minutes.
3. Broil or grill the marinated fish for about 4 minutes per side, basting regularly with the marinade.
4. Serve the grilled fish on a plate and top with the reserved marinade, thyme and chives.

Nutrition: Calories: 200; Total Fat: 8.1 g; Carbs: 5.5 g; Dietary Fiber: 0.5 g; Sugars: 2 g; Protein: 26.4 g; Cholesterol: 62 mg; Sodium: 91 mg

HEALTHY LOW-CARB GRILLED TURKEY

PREPARATION: 15 min.
COOKING TIME: 35 min.
SERVING: 12 People

Ingredients:
- 5 pounds turkey breast cutlets
- 3 tbsp. extra virgin olive oil
- 1-1/2 teaspoons garlic powder
- 1-1/2 teaspoons sweet paprika
- 2 tsp. crushed fennel seeds
- 1 teaspoon sea salt
- 1-1/2 teaspoons freshly ground black pepper

Directions:
1. Mix together garlic powder, paprika, fennel seeds, salt and pepper in a small bowl; rub the mixture over the turkey meat.
2. Add 3 tablespoons of olive oil to a skillet and heat over medium heat; add turkey meat and cook until browned on both sides.
3. Transfer the grilled turkey to a serving plate and let rest for about 5 minutes. Serve.

Nutrition: Calories: 258; Total Fat: 9.1 g; Carbs: 0.5 g; Dietary fiber: 0.2 g; Sugars: 0 g; Protein: 24 g; Cholesterol: 100 mg; Sodium: 334 mg

SATISFYING ARUGULA SALAD WITH FRUIT & CHICKEN

PREPARATION: 15 min.
COOKING TIME: 15 min.
SERVING: 1 Person

Ingredients:

- 1 tablespoon extra-virgin olive oil
- 100 grams chicken
- 2 cups arugula
- Strawberry or apple slices
- 1 tablespoon chopped red onion
- Pinch of salt & pepper
- Favorite dressing

Directions:

1. Brown the chicken in extra virgin olive oil. Prepare arugula and place sliced chicken on the arugula salad. Top with fruit and drizzle with dressing.

Nutrition: Calories: 281; Total Fat: 3.7 g; Carbs: 33.2 g; Dietary Fiber: 6.3 g; Sugars: 24.4 g; Protein: 30.7 g; Cholesterol: 77 mg; Sodium: 231 mg

TASTY COCONUT COD

PREPARATION: 25 min.
COOKING TIME: 10 min.
SERVING: 4 People

Ingredients:

- 24 ounces cod fillets, sliced into small strips
- 2 tablespoons coconut oil
- 1 cup finely shredded coconut
- 2 cups coconut milk
- 1 ½ cups coconut flour
- ¼ teaspoon sea salt
- 1 ½ teaspoon ginger powder

Directions:

1. Rinse and debone the fish fillets.
2. In a bowl, combine ginger powder, coconut flour and sea salt; set aside.
3. Add coconut milk to another bowl and set aside.
4. Add shredded coconut to another bowl and set aside.
5. Dip the fillets into coconut milk, then into the flour mixture, back into the milk, and finally into shredded coconut.
6. Add coconut oil to a skillet set over high heat; when melted and hot, add the fish fillets and cook for about 5 minutes per side or until cooked through.

Nutrition: Calories: 609; Total Fat: 44.3 g; Carbs: 13.2 g; Dietary Fiber: 6.4 g; Sugars: 5.7 g Protein: 43.1 g; Cholesterol: 34 mg; Sodium: 283 mg

SIDES AND SNACKS

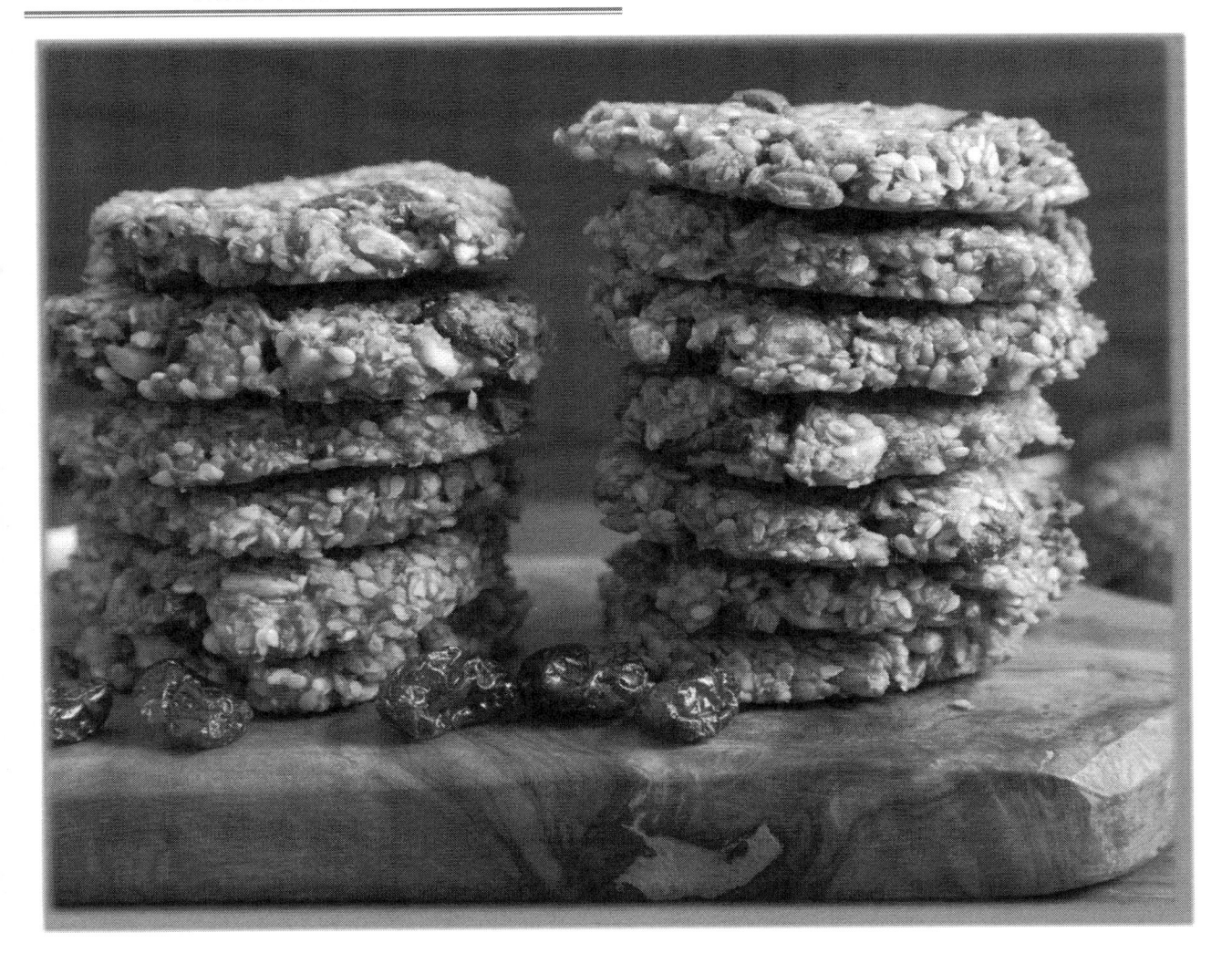

CITRUS SESAME COOKIES

PREPARATION: 15 min.
COOKING TIME: 10 min.
SERVING: 15 People

Ingredients:

- ¾ cup unsalted butter, at room temperature
- ½ cup sugar
- 1 egg
- 1 teaspoon vanilla extract
- 2 cups all-purpose flour
- 2 tablespoons toasted sesame seeds
- ½ teaspoon baking soda
- 1 teaspoon freshly grated lemon zest
- 1 teaspoon freshly grated orange zest

Directions:

1. In a large bowl and using a mixer, beat together the butter and sugar on high speed until thick and fluffy, about 3 minutes.
2. Add the egg and vanilla and beat to mix thoroughly, scraping down the sides of the bowl.
3. In a small bowl, stir together the flour, sesame seeds, baking soda, lemon zest, and orange zest.
4. Add the flour mixture to the butter mixture and stir until well blended.
5. Roll the dough into a long cylinder about 2 inches in diameter and wrap in plastic wrap. Refrigerate for 1 hour.
6. Preheat the oven to 350°F.
7. Line a baking sheet with parchment paper.
8. Cut the firm cookie dough into ½-inch-thick rounds and place them on the prepared baking sheet.
9. Bake for 10 to 12 minutes until lightly golden. Cool completely on wire racks.
10. Store in a sealed container in the refrigerator for up to 1 week, or in the freezer for up to 2 months.

Nutrients: Calories:150, Potassium:25mg, Phosphorous:29mg, Protein:2g, Sodium:5mg, Fat:9g

TRADITIONAL SPRITZ COOKIES

PREPARATION: 15 min.
COOKING TIME: 5 min.
SERVING: 24 People

Ingredients:

- 1 cup unsalted butter, at room temperature
- ½ cup sugar
- 1 egg
- 2 teaspoons vanilla extract
- 2½ cups all-purpose flour

Directions:

1. Preheat the oven to 400°F.
2. Line a baking sheet with parchment paper.
3. Beat in the egg and vanilla, scraping down the sides of the bowl.
4. Beat in the flour on low speed until blended.
5. Drop the cookies by the spoonful onto the prepared baking sheet.
6. Bake until firm and lightly golden, 5 to 7 minutes. Cool completely on a rack.
7. Store in a sealed container in a cool, dry place for up to 1 week.

Nutrients: Calories:271, Potassium:39mg Phosphorous: 40mg, Protein:3g, Sodium:11mg, Fat:16g

CLASSIC BAKING POWDER BISCUITS

PREPARATION: 15 min.
COOKING TIME: 12 min.
SERVING: 10 People

Ingredients:

- 2 cups all-purpose flour
- 1 tablespoon Phosphorus-Free Baking Powder (here)
- 1 tablespoon sugar
- ½ cup lard
- ½ cup water
- ¼ cup Homemade Rice Milk (here, or use unsweetened store-bought) or almond milk

Directions:

1. Preheat the oven to 350°F.
2. Line a baking sheet with parchment paper.
3. In a large bowl, stir together the flour, baking powder, and sugar.
4. Using your fingertips, rub the lard into the flour mixture until coarse crumbs form. Make a well in the center and pour in the water and rice milk. Use a fork to toss the mixture until it holds together as a dough. Do not overmix.
5. Pat the dough out on a lightly floured work surface until it is ½ inch thick.
6. Cut out 10 biscuits and place them on the prepared baking sheet.
7. Bake until light golden brown, 12 to 15 minutes.

Nutrients: Calories:190, Potassium:126mg, Phosphorous:27mg, Protein:3g, Sodium:45mg, Fat:10g

CRUNCHY CHICKEN SALAD WRAPS

PREPARATION: 15 min.
COOKING TIME:
SERVING: 4 People

Ingredients:

- 8 ounces cooked shredded chicken
- 1 scallion, white and green parts, chopped
- ½ cup halved seedless red grapes
- 1 celery stalk, chopped
- ¼ cup Low-Sodium Mayonnaise (here) or store-bought mayonnaise
- Pinch freshly ground black pepper
- 4 large lettuce leaves, butter, or red leaf

Directions:

1. In a medium bowl, stir together the chicken, scallion, grapes, celery, and mayonnaise until well mixed.
2. Season the mixture with pepper.
3. Spoon the chicken salad onto the lettuce leaves and serve.

Nutrients: Calories:110, Potassium:200mg, Phosphorous:117mg, Protein:13g, Sodium:61mg, Fat:13g

TASTY CHICKEN MEATBALLS

PREPARATION: 10 min.
COOKING TIME: 20 min.
SERVING: 6 People

Ingredients:

- ½ pound lean ground chicken
- ¼ cup breadcrumbs
- 1 scallion, white and green parts, chopped
- 1 egg, beaten
- 1 teaspoon minced garlic
- ¼ teaspoon freshly ground black pepper
- Pinch red pepper flakes

Directions:

1. Preheat the oven to 400°F.
2. In a large bowl, mix the chicken, breadcrumbs, scallion, egg, garlic, black pepper, and red pepper flakes.
3. Form the chicken mixture into 18 meatballs and place them on a baking sheet.
4. Bake the meatballs for about 25 minutes, turning several times, until golden brown.
5. Serve hot.

Nutrients: Calories: 85 Potassium: 200mg, Phosphorous: 91mg, Protein: 8g, Sodium: 67mg, Fat: 4g

HERB ROASTED CAULIFLOWER

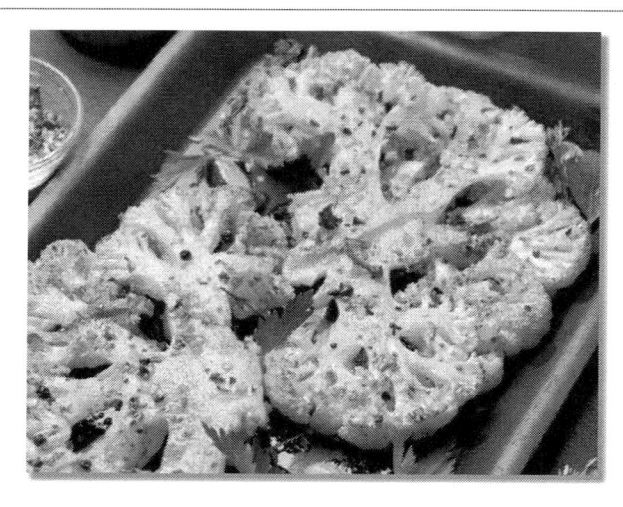

PREPARATION: 10 min.
COOKING TIME: 20 min.
SERVING: 4 People

Ingredients:

- 1 tablespoon olive oil, plus more for the pan
- 1 head cauliflower, cut in half and then into ½-inch-thick slices
- 1 teaspoon chopped fresh thyme
- 1 teaspoon chopped fresh chives
- ¼ teaspoon freshly ground black pepper

Directions:

1. Preheat the oven to 400°F.
2. Lightly coat a baking sheet with olive oil.
3. Toss the cauliflower, 1 tablespoon of olive oil, the thyme, chives, and pepper until well coated.
4. Spread the cauliflower on the prepared baking sheet.
5. Roast, turning once, until both sides are golden, about 20 minutes.

Nutrients: Calories:82, Potassium:200mg, Phosphorous:29mg, Protein:1g, Sodium:122mg, Fat:7g

SAUTEED BUTTERNUT SQUASH

PREPARATION: 10 min.
COOKING TIME: 20 min.
SERVING: 8 People

Ingredients:

- 1 tablespoon olive oil
- 4 cups peeled, seeded, 1-inch cubes butternut squash
- ½ sweet onion, chopped
- 1 teaspoon chopped fresh thyme
- Pinch freshly ground black pepper

Directions:

1. In a large skillet over medium-high heat, heat the olive oil.
2. Add the butternut squash and sauté until tender, about 15 minutes.
3. Add the onion and thyme, and sauté for 5 minutes.
4. Season with pepper and serve hot.

Nutrients: Calories: 45 Potassium: 200mg Phosphorous: 19mg Protein: 1g Sodium: 5mg, Fat: 1g

GERMAN BRAISED CABBAGE

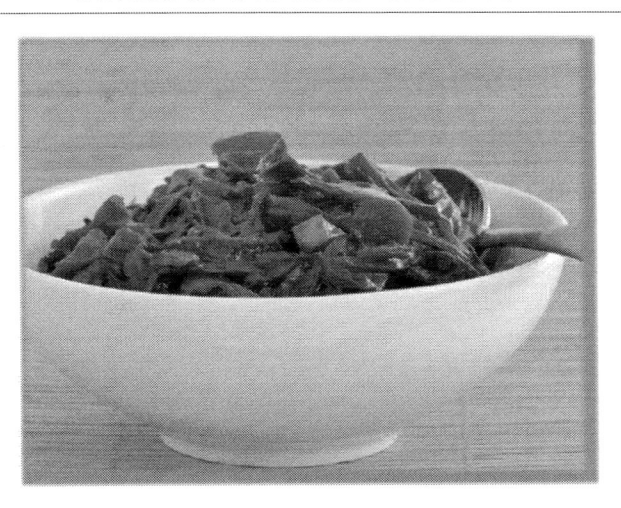

PREPARATION: 15 min.
COOKING TIME: 15 min.
SERVING: 4 People

Ingredients:

- 1 tablespoon olive oil
- 5 cups shredded red cabbage
- 1 pear, peeled, cored, and chopped
- ¼ large, sweet onion, chopped
- 3 tablespoons apple cider vinegar
- 1 tablespoon sugar
- ½ teaspoon caraway seed
- ½ teaspoon dry mustard

Directions:

1. In a large skillet over medium-high heat, heat the olive oil.
2. Add the cabbage, pear, and onion, and sauté until tender, about 10 minutes.
3. In a small bowl, stir together the vinegar, sugar, caraway seed, and mustard.
4. Pour the vinegar mixture into the cabbage and stir to combine. Cover and simmer the cabbage for 5 minutes.
5. Serve hot.

Nutrients: Calories: 62, Potassium: 161mg, Phosphorous: 23mg, Protein: 1g, Sodium: 14mg, Fat: 2g

WALNUT PILAF

PREPARATION: 5 min.
COOKING TIME: 30 min.
SERVING: 4 People

Ingredients:

- 1 teaspoon walnut oil
- ¼ sweet onion, chopped
- 1 cup white basmati rice
- 2 cups low-sodium chicken stock
- 1 tablespoon chopped toasted walnuts
- 2 tablespoons chopped fresh parsley

Directions:

1. In a large saucepan over low heat, heat the walnut oil.
2. Add the onion and rice, and sauté for 5 minutes.
3. Stir in the chicken stock, turn the heat to high, and bring the mixture to a boil. Cover, reduce the heat to low, and simmer until the liquid is absorbed, about 25 minutes.
4. Stir in the walnuts and parsley.
5. Serve hot.

Nutrients: Calories: 233, Potassium: 179mg, Phosphorous: 104mg, Protein: 6g, Sodium: 88mg, Fat: 5g

WILD MUSHROOM COUSCOUS

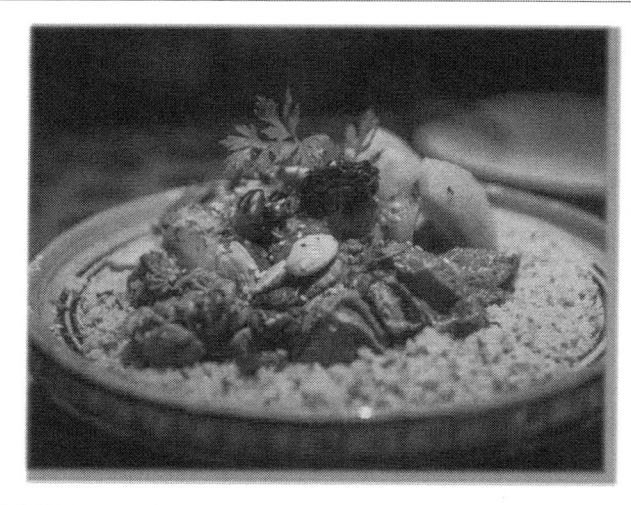

PREPARATION: 15 min.
COOKING TIME: 10 min.
SERVING: 4 People

Ingredients:

- 1 tablespoon olive oil
- 1 cup mixed wild mushrooms (shiitake, cremini, portobello, oyster, enoki)
- ¼ sweet onion, finely chopped
- 1 teaspoon minced garlic
- 1 tablespoon chopped fresh oregano
- 3½ cups water
- 10 ounces couscous

Directions:

1. In a large skillet over medium-high heat, heat the olive oil.
2. Add the mushrooms, onion, and garlic, and sauté until tender, about 6 minutes.
3. Stir in the oregano and water and bring the mixture to a boil.
4. Remove the saucepan from the heat and stir in the couscous.
5. Cover the saucepan and let it stand for 5 minutes.
6. Fluff the couscous with a fork and serve.

Nutrients: Calories: 237, Potassium: 165mg,

Phosphorous: 115mg, Protein: 8g, Sodium: 7mg, Fat: 3g

SPICY KALE CHIPS

PREPARATION: 20 min.
COOKING TIME: 25 min.
SERVING: 6 People

Ingredients:

- 2 cups kale
- 2 teaspoons olive oil
- ¼ teaspoon chili powder Pinch cayenne pepper

Directions:

1. Preheat the oven to 300°F.
2. Use parchment paper to line 2 baking pan and put aside.
3. Remove the stems from the kale and tear the leaves into 2-inch pieces.
4. Wash the kale and dry it completely.
5. Transfer the kale to a bowl and drizzle with olive oil.
6. Use your hands to toss the kale with the oil, taking care to coat each leaf evenly.
7. Season the kale with chili powder and cayenne pepper and toss to combine thoroughly.
8. Spread the seasoned kale in a single layer on each baking sheet. Do not overlap the leaves.
9. Bake the kale, rotating the pans once, for 20 to 25 minutes or until it is crisp and dry.
10. Take the trays from the oven and allow the chips to cool on the trays for 5 minutes.
11. Serve immediately.

Nutrition: Calories: 24; Fat: 2g; Carbohydrates: 2g; Phosphorus: 21mg; Potassium: 111mg; Sodium: 13g; Protein: 1g

CINNAMON TORTILLA CHIPS

PREPARATION: 15 min.
COOKING TIME: 10 min.
SERVING: 6 People

Ingredients:

- 2 teaspoons granulated sugar
- ½ teaspoon ground cinnamon
- Pinch ground nutmeg
- 3 (6-inch) flour tortillas
- Cooking spray, for coating the tortillas

Directions:

1. Preheat the oven to 350°F.
2. Line a baking sheet with parchment paper.
3. Stir together the sugar, cinnamon, and nutmeg in a small bowl.
4. Lay the tortillas on a surface previously cleaned and spray both sides of each lightly with cooking spray.
5. Sprinkle the cinnamon sugar evenly over both sides of each tortilla.
6. Cut the tortillas into 16 wedges each and place them on the baking sheet.
7. Bake the tortilla wedges, turning once, for about 10 minutes or until crisp.
8. Cool the chips and store in a sealed container at room temperature for up to 1 week.

Nutrition: Calories: 51; Fat: 1g; Carbohydrates: 9g; Phosphorus: 29mg; Potassium: 24mg; Sodium: 103mg; Protein: 1g

SWEET AND SPICY KETTLE CORN

PREPARATION: 1 min.
COOKING TIME: 5 min.
SERVING: 8 People

Ingredients:

- 3 tablespoons olive oil
- 1 cup popcorn kernels
- ½ cup brown sugar Pinch cayenne pepper

Directions:

1. Place a large pot with lid over medium heat and add the olive oil with a few popcorn kernels.
2. Shake the pot lightly until the popcorn kernels pop. Add sugar and rest of the kernels into the pot.
3. Pop the kernels with the lid on the pot, shaking constantly, until they are all popped.
4. Take the pot from the heat and transfer the popcorn to a large bowl.
5. Toss the popcorn with the cayenne pepper and serve.

Nutrition: Calories: 186; Fat: 6g; Carbohydrates: 30g; Phosphorus: 85mg; Potassium: 90mg; Sodium: 5mg; Protein: 3g

FIVE-SPICE CHICKEN LETTUCE WRAPS

PREPARATION: 30 min.
COOKING TIME: - min.
SERVING: 8 People

Ingredients:

- 6 ounces cooked chicken breast, chopped or preferably minced
- 1 scallion, green and white parts, chopped
- ½ red apple, cored and chopped
- ½ cup bean sprouts
- ¼ English cucumber, finely chopped Juice of 1 lime
- Zest of 1 lime
- 2 tablespoons chopped fresh cilantro
- ½ teaspoon Chinese five-spice powder
- 8 Boston lettuce leaves

Directions:

1. Get a big bowl now mix together the chicken, scallions, apple, bean sprouts, cucumber, lime juice, lime zest, cilantro, and five-spice powder.
2. Spoon the chicken mixture evenly among the 8 lettuce leaves.
3. Wrap the lettuce around the chicken mixture and serve.

Nutrition: Calories: 51; Fat: 2g; Carbohydrates: 2g; Phosphorus: 56mg; Potassium: 110mg; Sodium: 16mg; Protein: 7g

MERINGUE COOKIES

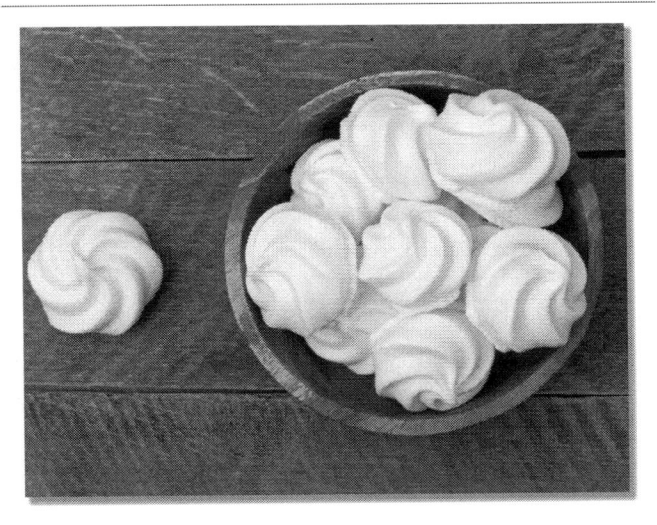

PREPARATION: 30 min.
COOKING TIME: 30 min.
SERVING: 24 People

Ingredients:

- 4 egg whites, at room temperature
- 1 cup granulated sugar
- 1 teaspoon pure vanilla extract
- 1 teaspoon almond extract

Directions:

1. Preheat the oven to 300°F.
2. Make use of parchment paper to line two baking pan; set aside.
3. Beat egg whites in a bowl of stainless steel with a whisk until stiff peaks develop.
4. Add some granulated sugar, 1 tablespoon at a time, beating well to incorporate after each addition, until all the sugar is used, and the meringue is thick and glossy.
5. Beat in the vanilla extract and almond extract.
6. Using a tablespoon, drop the meringue batter onto the baking sheets, spacing the cookies evenly.
7. Bake the cookies in an oven for approximately 30 minutes or until crisp.
8. Remove the cookies from the oven and let them cool on wire racks.
9. Store cookies in an airtight container with a lid at room temperature for up to 1 week.

Nutrition: Calories: 36; Fat: 0g; Carbohydrates: 8g; Phosphorus: 1mg; Potassium: 10mg; Sodium: 9mg; Protein: 1g

CORNBREAD

PREPARATION: 10 min.
COOKING TIME: 20 min.
SERVING: 10 People

Ingredients:

- Cooking spray, for greasing the baking dish
- 1¼ cups yellow cornmeal
- ¾ cup all-purpose flour
- 1 tablespoon Ener-G baking soda substitute
- ½ cup granulated sugar
- 2 eggs
- 1 cup unsweetened, unfortified rice milk
- 2 tablespoons olive oil

Directions:

1. Preheat the oven to 425°F.
2. Spray lightly an 8-by-8-inch baking dish with cooking spray; put aside.
3. In a medium bowl, stir together the cornmeal, flour, baking soda substitute, and sugar.
4. Whisk together the eggs, rice milk, and olive oil in a bowl until blended.
5. Combine the wet ingredients to the

dry ingredients and stir until well combined.
6. Move the batter into the baking dish and bake for close to 20 minutes or until golden and cooked through.
7. Serve warm.

Nutrition: Calories: 198; Fat: 5g; Carbohydrates: 34g; Phosphorus: 88mg; Potassium: 94mg; Sodium: 25mg; Protein: 4g

ROASTED RED PEPPER AND CHICKEN CROSTINI

PREPARATION: 10 min.
COOKING TIME: 5 min.
SERVING: 4 People

Ingredients:

- 2 tablespoons olive oil
- ½ teaspoon minced garlic
- 4 slices French bread
- 1 roasted red bell pepper, chopped
- 4 ounces cooked chicken breast, shredded
- ½ cup chopped fresh basil

Directions:
1. Preheat the oven to 400°F.
2. Line a baking sheet with aluminum foil.
3. Ensure olive oil and garlic are well mixed in a bowl.
4. Brush both sides of each piece of bread with the olive oil mixture.
5. Place the bread on the baking pan and toast in the oven, turning once, for about 5 minutes or until both sides are golden and crisp.
6. Stir together the red pepper, chicken, and basil in a pan
7. Top each toasted bread slice with the red pepper mixture and serve.

Nutrition: Calories: 184; Fat: 8g; Carbohydrates: 19g; Phosphorus: 87mg; Potassium: 152mg; Sodium: 175mg; Protein: 9g

BABA GHANOUSH

PREPARATION: 20 min.
COOKING TIME: 30 min.
SERVING: 6 People

Ingredients:

- 1 medium eggplant, halved and scored with a crosshatch pattern on the cut sides
- 1 tablespoon olive oil, plus extra for brushing
- 1 large, sweet onion, peeled and diced
- 2 garlic cloves, halved
- 1 teaspoon ground cumin
- 1 teaspoon ground coriander
- 1 tablespoon lemon juice
- Freshly ground black pepper

Directions:
1. Preheat the oven to 400°F.
2. Line 2 baking sheets with parchment paper.
3. Brush the eggplant halves with some olive oil and place them, cut side down, on 1 baking sheet.
4. Mix together the onion, garlic, 1 tablespoon olive oil, cumin, and coriander in a small bowl.
5. Spread the seasoned onions on the other baking sheet.
6. Put the two baking pans in the oven and allow onions to roast for about 25 minutes and the eggplant for 30 minutes, or until softened and browned.
7. Remove the vegetables from the oven and scrape the eggplant flesh into a bowl
8. Place the garlic and onions to a cutting board and chop coarsely; add to the eggplant

9. Stir in the lemon juice and pepper.
10. Serve warm or chilled.

Nutrition: Calories: 45; Fat: 2g; Carbohydrates: 6g; Phosphorus: 23mg; Potassium: 195mg; Sodium: 3mg; Protein: 1g

MIXED-GRAIN HOT CEREAL

PREPARATION: 10 min.
COOKING TIME: 25 min.
SERVING: 4 People

Ingredients:

- 2¼ cups water
- 1¼ cups vanilla rice milk
- 6 tablespoons uncooked bulgur
- 2 tablespoons uncooked whole buckwheat
- 1 cup peeled, sliced apple
- 6 tablespoons plain uncooked couscous
- ½ teaspoon ground cinnamon

Directions:

1. In a medium saucepan over medium-high heat, heat the water and milk.
2. Bring to a boil, and add the bulgur, buckwheat, and apple.
3. Lower the heat and allow to simmer, stirring occasionally, for 20 to 25 minutes or until the bulgur is tender.
4. Remove the saucepan from the heat and stir in the couscous and cinnamon.
5. Let the saucepan stand, covered, for 10 minutes, then fluff the cereal with a fork before serving.

Nutrition: Calories: 159; Fat: 1g; Carbohydrates: 34g; Phosphorus: 130mg; Potassium: 116mg; Sodium: 33mg; Protein: 4g

CINNAMON-NUTMEG BLUEBERRY MUFFINS

PREPARATION: 15 min.
COOKING TIME: 30 min.
SERVING: 10 People

Ingredients:

- 2 cups unsweetened rice milk
- 1 tablespoon apple cider vinegar
- 3½ cups all-purpose flour
- 1 cup granulated sugar
- 1 tablespoon Ener-G baking soda substitute
- 1 teaspoon ground cinnamon
- ½ teaspoon ground nutmeg Pinch ground ginger
- ½ cup canola oil
- 2 tablespoons pure vanilla extract
- 2½ cups fresh blueberries

Directions:

1. Preheat the oven to 375°F.
2. Muffin pan should be lined with paper liners; set aside.
3. In a small bowl, stir together the rice milk and vinegar; set aside for 10 minutes.
4. Stir together the flour, sugar, baking soda substitute, cinnamon, nutmeg, and ginger in a large bowl until well mixed. Add oil and vanilla to the milk mixture and stir until it blends.
5. Add the milk mixture to the dry ingredients and stir until well combined.
6. Fold in the blueberries. Spoon the

7. muffin batter evenly into the cups.
8. Bake the muffins for 25 to 30 minutes or until golden and a toothpick inserted in the center of a muffin comes out clean.
9. Allow the muffins to cool for 15 minutes before serving.

Nutrition: Calories: 331; Fat: 11g; Carbohydrates: 52g; Phosphorus: 90mg; Potassium: 89mg; Sodium: 35mg; Protein: 6g

FRUIT AND CHEESE BREAKFAST WRAP

PREPARATION: 10 min.
COOKING TIME: - min.
SERVING: 2 People

Ingredients:

- 2 (6-inch) flour tortillas
- 2 tablespoons plain cream cheese
- 1 apple, peeled, cored, and sliced thin
- 1 tablespoon honey

Directions:

1. Lay both tortillas on a clean work surface and spread 1 tablespoon of cream cheese onto each tortilla, leaving about ½ inch around the edges.
2. Arrange the apple slices on the cream cheese, just off the center of the tortilla on the side closest to you, leaving about 1½ inches on each side and 2 inches on the bottom.
3. Drizzle the apples lightly with honey.
4. Fold both the left and right edges of the tortillas into the center, laying the edge over the apples.
5. Taking the tortilla edge closest to you, fold it over the fruit and the side pieces. Roll the tortilla a bit away from you, creating a snug wrap.
6. Repeat with the second tortilla.

Nutrition: Calories: 188; Fat: 6g; Carbohydrates: 33g; Phosphorus: 73mg; Potassium: 136mg; Sodium: 177mg; Protein: 4g

EGG-IN-THE-HOLE

PREPARATION: 5 min.
COOKING TIME: 5 min.
SERVING: 2 People

Ingredients:

- 2 (½-inch-thick) slices Italian bread
- ¼ cup unsalted butter
- 2 eggs
- 2 tablespoons chopped fresh chives Pinch cayenne pepper
- Freshly ground black pepper

Directions:

1. Using a cookie cutter or a small glass, cut a 2-inch round from the center of each piece of bread.
2. Melt the butter in a large nonstick skillet over medium-high heat.
3. Place the bread in the skillet, toast it for 1 minute, and then flip the bread over.
4. Crack the eggs into the holes the center of the bread and cook for about 2 minutes or until the eggs are set and the bread is golden brown.
5. Top with chopped chives, cayenne pepper, and black pepper.
6. Cook the bread for another 2 minutes.
7. Transfer an egg-in-the-hole to each plate to serve.

Nutrition: Calories: 304; Fat: 29g; Carbohydrates: 12g; Phosphorus: 119mg; Potassium: 109mg; Sodium: 204mg; Protein: 9g

SKILLET-BAKED PANCAKE

PREPARATION: 15 min.
COOKING TIME: 20 min.
SERVING: 2 People

Ingredients:

- 2 eggs
- ½ cup unsweetened rice milk
- ½ cup all-purpose flour
- ¼ teaspoon ground cinnamon Pinch ground nutmeg
- Cooking spray, for greasing the skillet

Directions:

1. Preheat the oven to 450°F
2. Whisk the eggs and rice milk together in a medium bowl.
3. Stir in the flour, cinnamon, and nutmeg until blended but still slightly lumpy, but do not overmix.
4. Spray with a cooking spray a 9-inch ovenproof skillet and place the skillet in the preheated oven for 5 minutes.
5. Remove the skillet carefully and pour the pancake batter into the skillet.
6. Return the skillet to the oven and bake the pancake for approximately 20 minutes or until the edges are puffed up and crispy.
7. Cut the pancake into halves to serve.
8. Dialysis modification: If you need additional protein in this dish, whisk in an extra egg white. There will be no change in texture nor taste.

Nutrition: Calories: 161; Fat: 1g; Carbohydrates: 30g; Phosphorus: 73mg; Potassium: 106mg; Sodium: 79mg; Protein: 7g

TUNA CUCUMBER BITES

PREPARATION: 5 min.
COOKING TIME: -
SERVING: 2 People

Ingredients:

- Tuna, light, canned – 1 can
- Tofu, soft - .33 cup
- Onion, thinly sliced - .33 cup
- Cucumber, sliced – 1
- Black pepper, ground - .25 teaspoon
- Garlic powder - .25 teaspoon

Directions:

1. Place the black pepper, powder, and soft tofu garlic together in a bowl and then mash them together with a fork until the tofu is broken down.
2. Drain the light tuna and then add it to the tofu mixture along with the thinly sliced onion and stir the mixture together until it is fully combined.
3. Slice your cucumber and then place the slices on a plate and top the slices off with the tuna mixture. Serve the tuna slices immediately.

Nutrition: Calories:118 Potassium:370 mg Phosphorous:181mg Protein:19g Sodium:210mg, Fat:2g

CINNAMON CANDIED ALMONDS

PREPARATION: 2 min.
COOKING TIME: 7 min.
SERVING: 2 People

Ingredients:

- Truvia sweetener – .25 cup
- Almonds, raw – .5 cup
- Cinnamon – 1 teaspoon
- Water – 1 tablespoon
- Vanilla extract - .25 teaspoon

Directions:

1. Place a skillet over medium heat and allow it to warm up. Once the skillet is hot, add in the Truvia sweetener, water, cinnamon, and vanilla extract. Using a spoon, combine the mixture and continue to stir it while it melts.

2. Once the Truvia mixture has completely melted, add in the almonds and stir to coat the almonds completely. Continue to stir and cook until the mixture begins to crystallize to the almonds, and then remove it from the heat.

3. Allow the almonds to sit for two to three minutes, and then use a spatula to break them apart before they stick together.

4. Allow the almonds to cool before serving them.

Nutrition: Calories:212, Potassium:268 mg, Phosphorous:173mg, Protein:7g, Sodium:1mg, Fat:17g

FISH AND SEAFOODS ENTRÉES

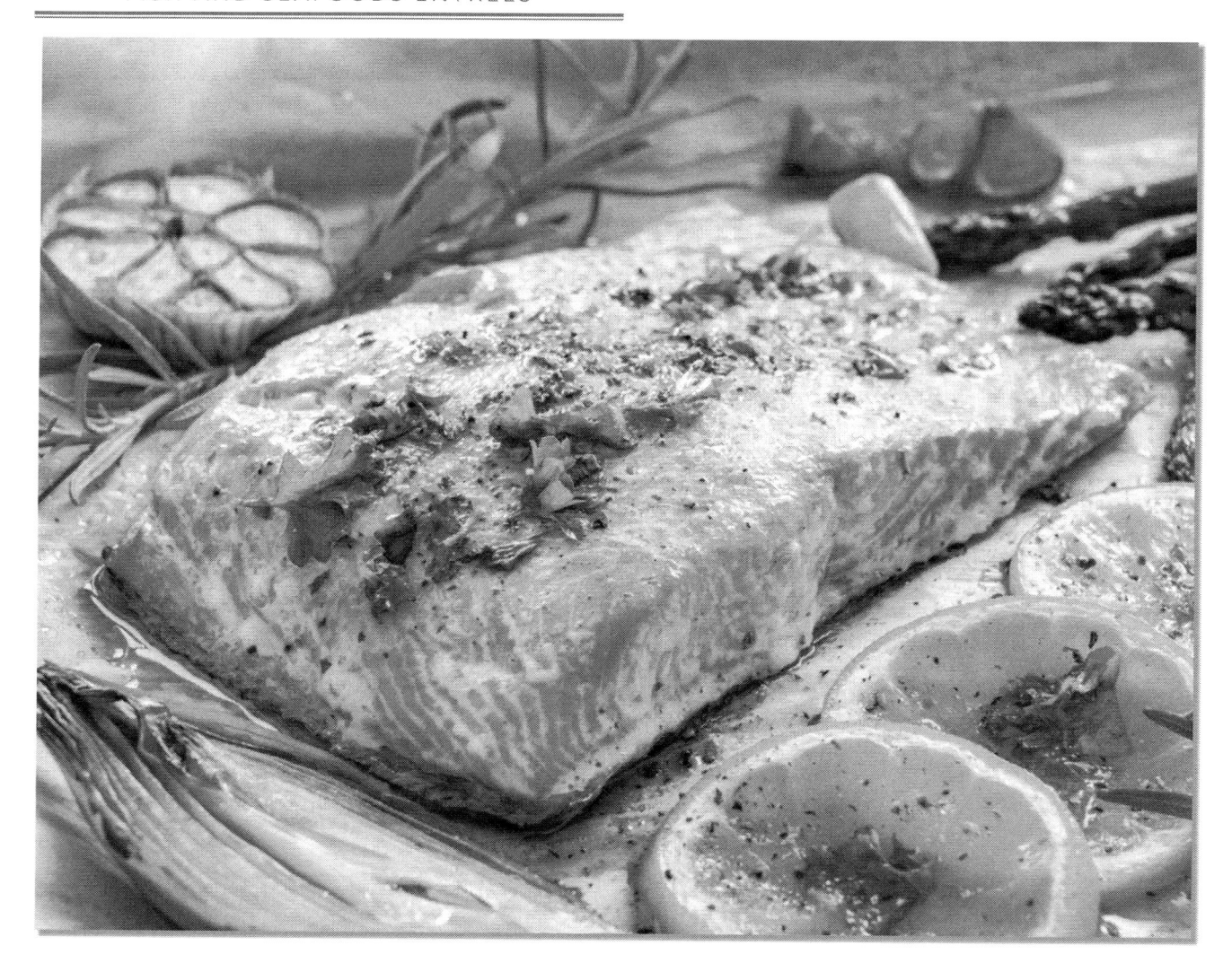

GRILLED SHRIMP WITH CUCUMBER LIME SALSA

PREPARATION: 15 min.
COOKING TIME: 10 min.
SERVING: 4 People

Ingredients:

- 2 tablespoons olive oil
- 6 ounces large shrimp (16 to 20 count), peeled and deveined, tails left on
- 1 teaspoon minced garlic
- ½ cup chopped English cucumber
- ½ cup chopped mango
- Zest of 1 lime
- Juice of 1 lime
- Freshly ground black pepper
- Lime wedges for garnish

Directions:

1. Soak 4 wooden skewers in water for 30 minutes.
2. Preheat the barbecue to medium-high heat.
3. In a large bowl, toss together the olive oil, shrimp, and garlic.
4. Thread the shrimp onto the skewers, about 4 shrimp per skewer.
5. In a small bowl, stir together the cucumber, mango, lime zest, and lime juice, and season the salsa lightly with pepper. Set aside.
6. Grill the shrimp for about 10 minutes, turning once or until the shrimp is opaque and cooked through.
7. Season the shrimp lightly with pepper.
8. Serve the shrimp on the cucumber salsa with lime wedges on the side.

Nutrition: Calories: 120 Potassium: 129mg, Phosphorous: 91mg, Protein: 9g, Sodium: 60mg, Fat: 8g

SHRIMP SCAMPI LINGUINE

PREPARATION: 15 min.
COOKING TIME: 10 min.
SERVING: 4 People

Ingredients:

- 4 ounces uncooked linguine
- 1 teaspoon olive oil
- 2 teaspoons minced garlic
- 4 ounces shrimp, peeled, deveined, and chopped
- ½ cup dry white wine
- Juice of 1 lemon
- 1 tablespoon chopped fresh basil
- ½ cup heavy (whipping) cream
- Freshly ground black pepper

Directions:

1. Cook the linguine according to the package instructions; drain and set aside.
2. In a large skillet over medium heat, heat the olive oil
3. Sauté the garlic and shrimp for about 6 minutes or until the shrimp is opaque and just cooked through.
4. Add the wine, lemon juice, and basil, and cook for 5 minutes.
5. Stir in the cream and simmer for 2 minutes more.
6. Add the linguine to the skillet and toss to coat.
7. Divide the pasta onto 4 plates to serve.

Nutrition: Calories: 219, Potassium: 155mg, Phosphorous: 119mg, Protein: 12g, Sodium: 42mg, Fat:7g

CRAB CAKES WITH LIME SALSA

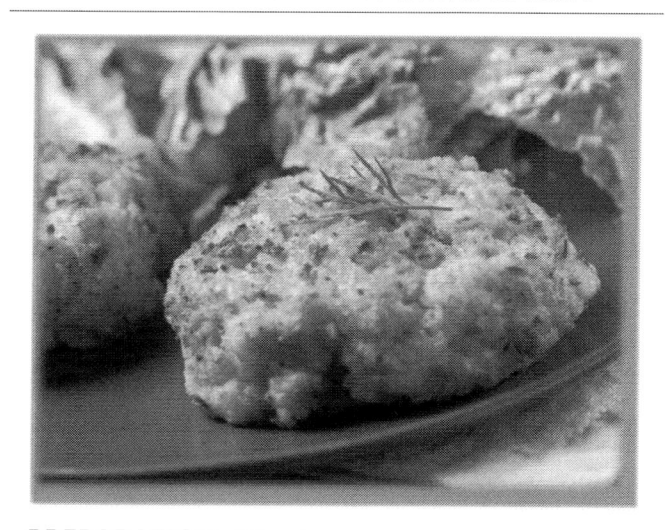

PREPARATION: 20 min.
COOKING TIME: 20 min.
SERVING: 4 People

Ingredients:

FOR THE SALSA

- ½ English cucumber, diced
- 1 lime, chopped
- ½ cup boiled and chopped red bell pepper
- 1 teaspoon chopped fresh cilantro
- Freshly ground black pepper

FOR THE CRAB CAKES

- 8 ounces queen crab meat
- ¼ cup breadcrumbs
- 1 small egg
- ¼ cup boiled and chopped red bell pepper
- 1 scallion, both green and white parts, minced
- 1 tablespoon chopped fresh parsley
- Splash hot sauce
- Olive oil spray, for the pan

Directions:

TO MAKE THE SALSA

1. In a small bowl, stir together the cucumber, lime, red pepper, and cilantro.
2. Season with pepper; set aside.

TO MAKE THE CRAB CAKES

1. In a medium bowl, mix together the crab, breadcrumbs, egg, red pepper, scallion, parsley, and hot sauce until it holds together. Add more breadcrumbs, if necessary.
2. Form the crab mixture into 4 patties and place them on a plate.
3. Refrigerate the crab cakes for 1 hour to firm them.
4. Spray a large skillet generously with olive oil spray and place it over medium-high heat.
5. Cook the crab cakes in batches, turning, for about 5 minutes per side or until golden brown.
6. Serve the crab cakes with the salsa.

Nutrition: Calories: 115, Potassium: 200mg, Phosphorous: 110mg, Protein:16g, Sodium:421mg, Fat:2g

SEAFOOD CASSEROLE

PREPARATION: 20 min.
COOKING TIME: 45 min.
SERVING: 6 People

Ingredients:

- 2 cups eggplant, peeled and diced into 1-inch pieces
- Butter, for greasing the baking dish
- 1 tablespoon olive oil
- ½ small, sweet onion, chopped
- 1 teaspoon minced garlic
- 1 celery stalk, chopped
- ½ red bell pepper, boiled and chopped
- 3 tablespoons freshly squeezed lemon juice
- 1 teaspoon hot sauce
- ¼ teaspoon Creole Seasoning Mix (here)
- ½ cup white rice, uncooked
- 1 large egg
- 4 ounces cooked shrimp
- 6 ounces queen crab meat

Directions:

1. Preheat the oven to 350°F.
2. In a small saucepan filled with water over medium-high heat, boil the eggplant for 5 minutes. Drain and set aside in a large bowl.
3. Grease a 9-by-13-inch baking dish with butter and set aside.
4. In a large skillet over medium heat, heat the olive oil.
5. Sauté the onion, garlic, celery, and bell pepper for about 4 minutes or until they are tender.
6. Add the sautéed vegetables to the eggplant, along with the lemon juice, hot sauce, Creole seasoning, rice, and egg.
7. Stir to combine
8. Fold in the shrimp and crab meat.
9. Spoon the casserole mixture into the casserole dish, patting down the top.
10. Bake for 25 to 30 minutes or until the casserole is heated through and the rice is tender
11. Serve warm.

Nutrition: Calories:118, Potassium:199mg, Phosphorous:102mg, Protein:12g, Sodium:235mg, Fat:4g

SWEET GLAZED SALMON

PREPARATION: 10 min.
COOKING TIME: 10 min. plus 1-hour chilling time
SERVING: 4 People

Ingredients:

- 2 tablespoons honey
- 1 teaspoon lemon zest
- ½ teaspoon freshly ground black pepper
- 4 (3-ounce) salmon fillets
- 1 tablespoon olive oil
- ½ scallion, white and green parts, chopped

Directions:

1. In a small bowl, stir together the honey, lemon zest, and pepper.
2. Wash the salmon and pat dry with paper towels
3. Rub the honey mixture all over each fillet.
4. In a large skillet over medium heat, heat the olive oil.

5. Add the salmon fillets and cook the salmon for about 10 minutes, turning once, or until it is lightly browned and just cooked through.
6. Serve topped with chopped scallion.

Nutrition: Calories: 240, Potassium: 317mg, Phosphorous: 205mg, Protein: 17g, Sodium: 51mg, Fat: 15g

HERB-CRUSTED BAKED HADDOCK

PREPARATION: 10 min.
COOKING TIME: 20 min.
SERVING: 4 People

Ingredients:

- ½ cup breadcrumbs
- 3 tablespoons chopped fresh parsley
- 1 tablespoon lemon zest
- 1 teaspoon chopped fresh thyme
- ¼ teaspoon freshly ground black pepper
- 1 tablespoon melted unsalted butter
- 12-ounces haddock fillets, deboned and skinned

Directions:

1. Preheat the oven to 350°F.
2. In a small bowl, stir together the breadcrumbs, parsley, lemon zest, thyme, and pepper until well combined.
3. Add the melted butter and toss until the mixture resembles coarse crumbs
4. Place the haddock on a baking sheet and spoon the bread crumb mixture on top, pressing down firmly.
5. Bake the haddock in the oven for about 20 minutes or until the fish is just cooked through and flakes off in chunks when pressed.

Nutrition: Calories: 143, Potassium: 285mg, Phosphorous: 216mg, Protein:16g, Sodium: 281mg, Fat:4g

SHORE LUNCH—STYLE SOLE

PREPARATION: 20 min.
COOKING TIME: 10 min.
SERVING: 4 People

Ingredients:

- ¼ cup all-purpose flour
- ¼ teaspoon freshly ground black pepper
- 12 ounces sole fillets, deboned and skinned
- 2 tablespoons olive oil
- 1 scallion, both green and white parts, chopped
- Lemon wedges, for garnish

Directions:

1. In a large plastic freezer bag, shake together the flour and pepper to combine.
2. Add the fish fillets to the flour and shake to coat.
3. In a large skillet over medium-high heat, heat the olive oil.
4. When the oil is hot, add the fish fillets and fry for about 10 minutes, turning once, or until they are golden and cooked through.
5. Remove the fish from the oil onto paper towels to drain.
6. Serve topped with chopped scallions and a squeeze of lemon.

Nutrition: Calories: 148, Potassium: 148mg,

Phosphorous: 223m,g Protein: 11g, Sodium: 242mg, Fat:8g

BAKED COD WITH CUCUMBER-DILL SALSA

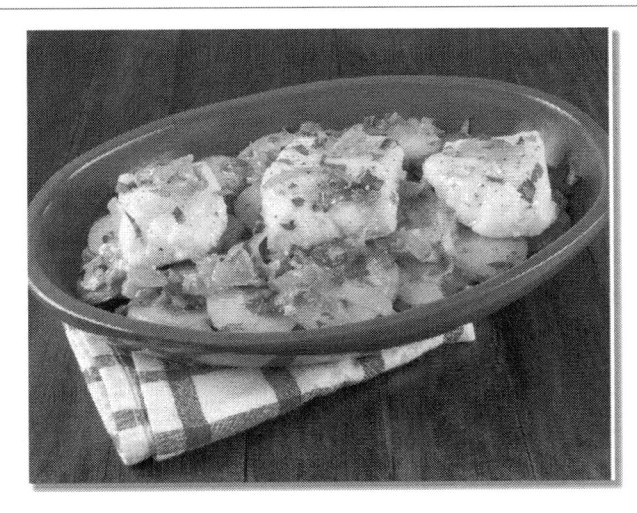

PREPARATION: 20 min.
COOKING TIME: 10 min.
SERVING: 4 People

Ingredients:

FOR THE CUCUMBER SALSA

- ½ English cucumber, chopped
- 2 tablespoons chopped fresh dill
- Juice of 1 lime
- Zest of 1 lime
- ¼ cup boiled and minced red bell pepper
- ½ teaspoon granulated sugar

FOR THE FISH

- 12 ounces cod fillets, deboned and cut into 4 servings
- Juice of 1 lemon
- ½ teaspoon freshly ground black pepper
- 1 teaspoon olive oil

Directions:

TO MAKE THE CUCUMBER SALSA

1. In a small bowl, mix together the cucumber, dill, lime juice, lime zest, red pepper, and sugar; set aside.

TO MAKE THE FISH

1. Preheat the oven to 350°F.
2. Place the fish on a pie plate and squeeze the lemon juice evenly over the fillets.
3. Sprinkle with pepper and drizzle the olive oil evenly over the fillets.
4. Bake the fish for about 6 minutes or until it flakes easily with a fork.
5. Transfer the fish to 4 plates and serve topped with cucumber salsa.

Nutrition: Calories:110, Potassium:275mg, Phosphorous:120mg, Protein:20g, Sodium:67mg, Fat:2g

CILANTRO-LIME FLOUNDER

PREPARATION: 20 min.
COOKING TIME: 5
SERVING: 4 People

Ingredients:

- ¼ cup Homemade Mayonnaise (here)
- Juice of 1 lime
- Zest of 1 lime
- ½ cup chopped fresh cilantro
- 4 (3-ounce) flounder fillets
- Freshly ground black pepper

Directions:

1. Preheat the oven to 400°F.
2. In a small bowl, stir together the mayonnaise, lime juice, lime zest, and cilantro.
3. Place 4 pieces of foil, about 8 by 8 inches square, on a clean work surface.
4. Place a flounder fillet in the center of each square
5. Top the fillets evenly with the mayonnaise mixture.
6. Season the flounder with pepper.
7. Bake the fish 4 to 5 minutes.
8. Unfold the packets and serve.

Nutrition: Calories:92, Potassium:137mg, Phosphorous:208mg, Protein:12g, Sodium:267mg, Fat:4g

HERB PESTO TUNA

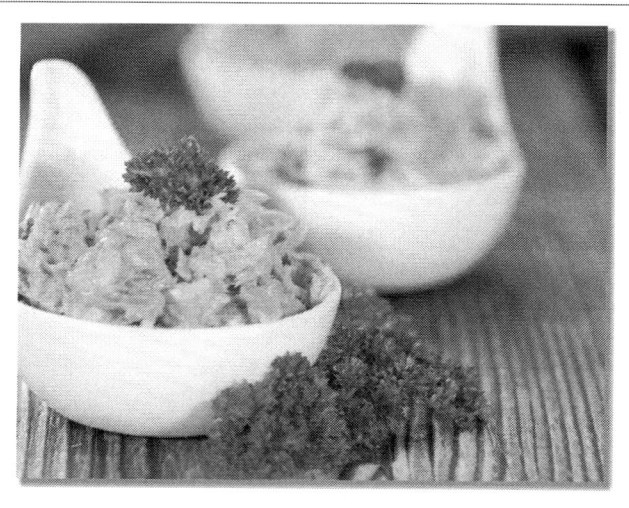

PREPARATION: 10 min.
COOKING TIME: 10 min.
SERVING: 4 People

Ingredients:

- 4 (3-ounce) yellowfin tuna fillets
- 1 teaspoon olive oil
- Freshly ground black pepper
- ¼ cup Herb Pesto (see here)
- 1 lemon, cut into 8 thin slices

Directions:

1. Heat the barbecue to medium-high.
2. Drizzle the fish with the olive oil and season each fillet with pepper.
3. Cook the fish on the barbecue for 4 minutes.
4. Turn the fish over and top each piece with the herb pesto and lemon slices.
5. Grill for 5 to 6 minutes more or until the tuna is cooked to medium-well

Nutrition: Calories: 103, Potassium: 374mg, Phosphorous: 236mg, Protein: 21g, Sodium: 38mg, Fat:2g

GRILLED CALAMARI WITH LEMON AND HERBS

PREPARATION: 10 min. plus 1-hour marinating
COOKING TIME: 3 min.
SERVING: 4 People

Ingredients:

- 2 tablespoons olive oil
- 2 tablespoons freshly squeezed lemon juice
- 1 tablespoon chopped fresh parsley
- 1 tablespoon chopped fresh oregano
- 2 teaspoons minced garlic
- Pinch sea salt
- Pinch freshly ground black pepper
- ½ pound cleaned calamari
- Lemon wedges, for garnish

Directions:

1. In large bowl, stir together the olive oil, lemon juice, parsley, oregano, garlic, salt, and pepper.
2. Add the calamari to the bowl and stir to coat
3. Cover the bowl and refrigerate the calamari for 1 hour to marinate.
4. Preheat the barbecue to medium-high.
5. Grill the calamari, turning once, until firm and opaque, about 3 minutes total.
6. Serve with lemon wedges.

Nutrition: Calories: 81, Potassium: 160mg, Phosphorous: 128mg, Protein: 3g, Sodium: 67mg, Fat: 7g

LEMONY HADDOCK

PREPARATION: 10 min. plus 1-hour marinating
COOKING TIME: 20 min.
SERVING: 1 Person

Ingredients:

- 1 tablespoon melted unsalted butter
- 12-ounces haddock fillets, deboned and skinned
- ½ cup breadcrumbs
- 3 tablespoons chopped fresh parsley
- 1 tablespoon lemon zest
- 1 teaspoon chopped fresh thyme
- ¼ teaspoon black pepper (ground)

Directions:

1. Preheat the oven to 350°F.
2. In a mixing bowl, add breadcrumbs, parsley, lemon zest, thyme, and pepper. Combine to mix well.
3. Add butter and combine until you get crumbles.
4. Take a baking sheet and place haddock on it. Add crumb mixture on top.
5. Bake for 18-20 minutes until evenly brown from top.
6. Serve warm.

Nutrition: Calories: 183 Potassium: 305mg, Phosphorous: 233mg, Protein: 16g, Sodium: 316mg, Fat:4g

GLAZED SALMON

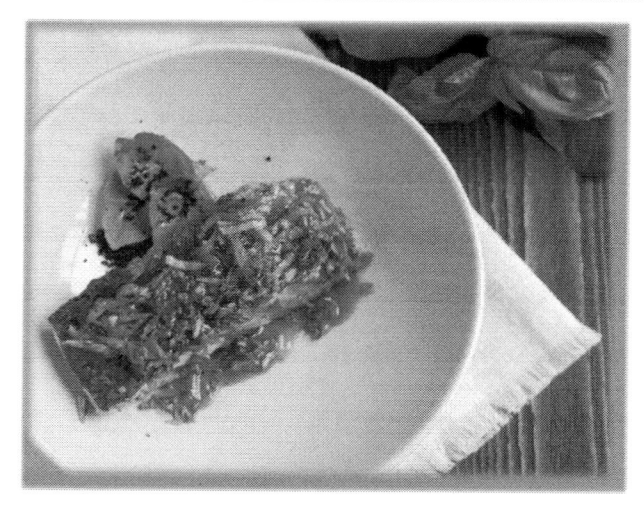

PREPARATION: 10 min.
COOKING TIME: 10 min.
SERVING: 1 Person

Ingredients:

- 4 (3-ounce) salmon fillets
- 1 tablespoon olive oil
- 2 tablespoons honey
- 1 teaspoon lemon zest
- ½ teaspoon Black pepper (ground), to taste
- ½ scallion, chopped

Directions:

1. Pat dry salmon with paper towels.
2. In a mixing bowl, add honey, lemon zest, and pepper. Combine to mix well.
3. Add salmon and coat evenly.
4. Take a medium saucepan or skillet, add oil. Heat over medium heat.
5. Add salmon and stir-cook until light brown and cooked well, for about 8-10 minutes. Flip in between.
6. Serve warm with scallions on top.

Nutrition: Calories: 238, Potassium: 348mg, Phosphorous: 220mg, Protein: 16g, Sodium: 74mg, Fat: 13g

TUNA CASSEROLE

PREPARATION: 15 min.
COOKING TIME: 35
SERVING: 1 People

Ingredients:

- ½ cup Cheddar cheese, shredded
- 2 tomatoes, chopped
- 7 oz tuna filet, chopped
- 1 teaspoon ground coriander
- ½ teaspoon salt
- 1 teaspoon olive oil
- ½ teaspoon dried oregano

Directions:

1. Brush the casserole mold with olive oil.
2. Mix together chopped tuna fillet with dried oregano and ground coriander.
3. Place the fish in the mold and flatten well to get the layer.
4. Then add chopped tomatoes and shredded cheese.
5. Cover the casserole with foil and secure the edges.
6. Bake the meal for 35 minutes at 3550 F.

Nutrition: Calories: 260 Potassium: 64mg, Phosphorous: 56mg, Protein:14.6g, Sodium: 29mg, Fat: 21.5g

OREGANO SALMON WITH CRUNCHY CRUST

PREPARATION: 10 min.
COOKING TIME: 2 hours
SERVING: 2 People

Ingredients:

- 8 oz salmon fillet
- 2 tablespoons panko breadcrumbs
- 1 oz Parmesan, grated
- 1 teaspoon dried oregano
- 1 teaspoon sunflower oil

Directions:

1. In the mixing bowl combine panko breadcrumbs, Parmesan, and dried oregano.
2. Sprinkle the salmon with olive oil and coat in the breadcrumb's mixture.
3. After this, line the baking tray with baking paper.
4. Place the salmon in the tray and transfer to the oven preheated at 3850 F.
5. Bake the salmon for 25 minutes.

Nutrition: Calories: 245Kcal; Fat 12.8g; Phosphorus: 30mg; Potassium: 67mg; Sodium: 31mg; Fiber 0.6g; Carbs: 5.9g; Protein: 27.5g.

SARDINE FISH CAKES

PREPARATION: 10 min.
COOKING TIME: 10 min.
SERVING: 1 Person

Ingredients:

- 11 oz sardines, canned, drained
- 1/3 cup shallot, chopped
- 1 teaspoon chili flakes
- ½ teaspoon salt
- 2 tablespoon wheat flour, whole grain
- 1 egg, beaten
- 1 tablespoon chives, chopped
- 1 teaspoon olive oil
- 1 teaspoon butter

Directions:

1. Put the butter in the skillet and melt it.
2. Add shallot and cook it until translucent.
3. After this, transfer the shallot in the mixing bowl.
4. Add sardines, chili flakes, salt, flour, egg, chives, and mix up until smooth with the help of the fork.
5. Make the medium size cakes and place them in the skillet.
6. Add olive oil.
7. Roast the fish cakes for 3 minutes from each side over the medium heat.
8. Dry the cooked fish cakes with the paper towel if needed and transfer in the serving plates.

Nutrition: Calories: 221; Fat: 12.2; Phosphorus: 36mg; Potassium: 194mg; Sodium: 31mg; Fiber 0.1; Carbs 5.4; Protein 21.3g

CAJUN CATFISH

PREPARATION: 10 min.
COOKING TIME: 10 min.
SERVING: 1 Person

Ingredients:

- 16 oz catfish steaks (4 oz each fish steak)
- 1 tablespoon Cajun spices
- 1 egg, beaten
- 1 tablespoon sunflower oil

Directions:

1. Heat oil in a pan.
2. Meanwhile, dip every catfish steak in the beaten egg and coat in Cajun spices.
3. Place the fish steaks in the hot oil and roast them for 4 minutes from each side.
4. The cooked catfish steaks should have a light brown crust.

Nutrition: Calories: 263; Fat: 16.7; Phosphorus: 39mg; Potassium: 74mg; Sodium: 20mg; Fiber: 0; Carbs: 0.1; Protein: 26.3g.

POACHED GENNARO/SEABASS WITH RED PEPPERS

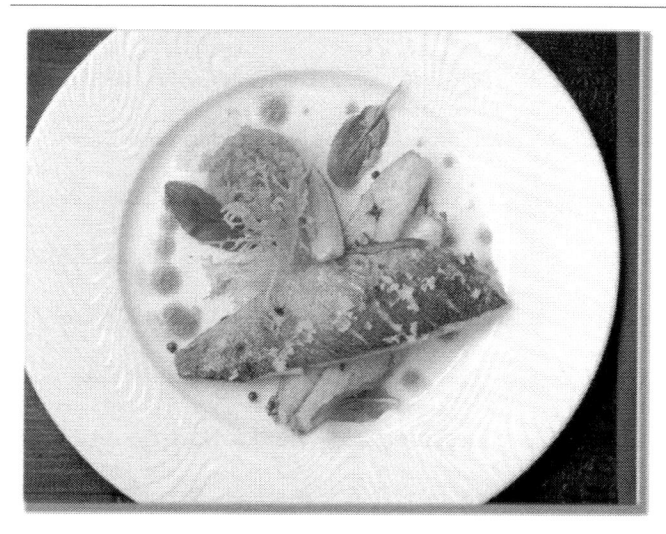

PREPARATION: 10 min.
COOKING TIME: 40 min.
SERVING: 1 People

Ingredients:

- 2 red peppers, trimmed
- 11 oz Gennaro/seabass, trimmed
- 1 teaspoon salt
- ½ teaspoon ground black pepper
- 2 tablespoons butter
- 1 lemon

Directions:

1. Remove the seeds from red peppers and cut them into wedges.
2. Then line the baking tray with parchment and arrange red peppers in a layer.
3. Rub Gennaro/seabass with ground black pepper and salt and place it on the peppers.
4. Then add butter.
5. Cut the lemon on the halves and squeeze the juice over the fish.
6. Bake the fish for 40 minutes at 3500 F.

Nutrition: Calories: 148, Fat: 10.3, Phosphorus:

36mg; Potassium: 194mg; Sodium: 31mg; Fiber:1.2, Carbs: 7.3, Protein: 8.5g.

4-INGREDIENTS SALMON FILLET

PREPARATION: 5 min.
COOKING TIME: 25 min.
SERVING: 1 Person

Ingredients:

- 4 oz salmon fillet
- ½ teaspoon salt
- 1 teaspoon sesame oil
- ½ teaspoon sage

Directions:

1. Rub the fillet with salt and sage.
2. Place the fish in the tray and sprinkle it with sesame oil.
3. Cook the fish for 25 minutes at 3650 F.
4. Flip the fish carefully onto another side after 12 minutes of cooking.

Nutrition: Calories: 191; Phosphorus: 30mg; Potassium: 74mg; Sodium: 30mg; Fat 11.6; Fiber: 0.1; Carbs: 0.2; Protein: 22g.

OREGANO GRILLED CALAMARI

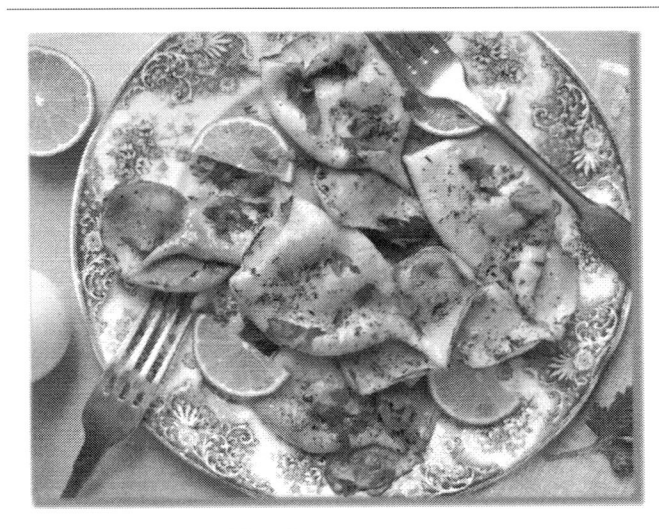

PREPARATION: 10 min.
COOKING TIME: 10 min.
SERVING: 1 Person

Ingredients:

- 2 teaspoons garlic, minced
- Pinch sea salt
- 2 tablespoons olive oil
- 2 tablespoons lemon juice
- 1 tablespoon chopped fresh parsley
- 1 tablespoon chopped fresh oregano
- Pinch black pepper (ground)
- ½ pound cleaned calamari
- Lemon wedges

Directions:

1. In a mixing bowl, add olive oil, lemon juice, parsley, oregano, garlic, salt, and pepper. Combine to mix well.
2. Add calamari and combine again. Refrigerate to marinate for 1 hour.
3. Preheat grill over medium heat setting.
4. Grease grates with some oil.
5. Grill calamari for 3 minutes, until evenly cooked. Turn halfway through.
6. Serve warm with some lemon wedges.

Nutrition: Calories: 103; Fat: 6g; Phosphorus: 130mg; Potassium: 176mg; Sodium: 73mg; Carbohydrates: 2g; Protein: 4g.

BAKED SHRIMP CRABS

PREPARATION: 10 min.
COOKING TIME: 30 min.
SERVING: 1 Person

Ingredients:

- 4 tablespoons green pepper, chopped
- 2 tablespoons green onions, chopped
- 1 cup celery, chopped
- 1 cup crabmeat, cooked (boiled)
- 1 cup shrimp, cooked (boiled)
- ½ cup frozen green peas, thawed
- ½ teaspoon black pepper
- ½ cup mayonnaise
- 1 cup breadcrumbs

Directions:

1. Preheat the oven to 375°F. Grease a casserole dish with some cooking spray.
2. In a mixing bowl, add all ingredients except breadcrumbs. Combine to mix well.
3. Add the mixture in a casserole dish and bake for 30 minutes until evenly brown.
4. Serve warm.

Nutrition: Calories: 268; Fat: 7g; Phosphorus: 159mg; Potassium: 287mg; Sodium: 466mg; Carbohydrates: 21g; Protein: 17g.

SALMON STUFFED PASTA

PREPARATION: 10 min.
COOKING TIME: 35 min.
SERVING: 4 Person

Ingredients:
- 24 jumbo pasta shells, boiled
- 1 cup coffee creamer

Filling:
- 2 eggs, beaten
- 2 cups creamed cottage cheese
- ¼ cup chopped onion
- 1 red bell pepper, diced
- 2 teaspoons dried parsley
- ½ teaspoon lemon peel
- 1 can salmon, drained

Dill Sauce:
- 1 ½ teaspoon butter
- 1 ½ teaspoon flour
- 1/8 teaspoon pepper
- 1 tablespoon lemon juice
- 1 ½ cup coffee creamer
- 2 teaspoons dried dill weed

Directions:

1. Beat the egg with the cream cheese and all the other filling ingredients in a bowl.
2. Divide the filling and fill in the pasta shells and place the shells in a 9x13 baking dish.
3. Pour the coffee creamer around the stuffed shells then cover with a foil.
4. Bake the shells for 30 minutes at 3500 F.
5. Meanwhile, whisk all the ingredients for dill sauce in a saucepan.
6. Stir for 5 minutes, until it thickens.
7. Pour this sauce over the baked pasta shells.
8. Serve warm.

Nutrition: Calories: 268; Total Fat 4.8g; Cholesterol: 27mg; Sodium: 86mg; Total Carbohydrate: 42.6g; Dietary Fiber: 2.1g; Sugars: 2.4g; Protein: 11.5g; Calcium: 27mg; Phosphorous: 314mg; Potassium: 181mg.

MEAT AND POULTRY ENTRÉES

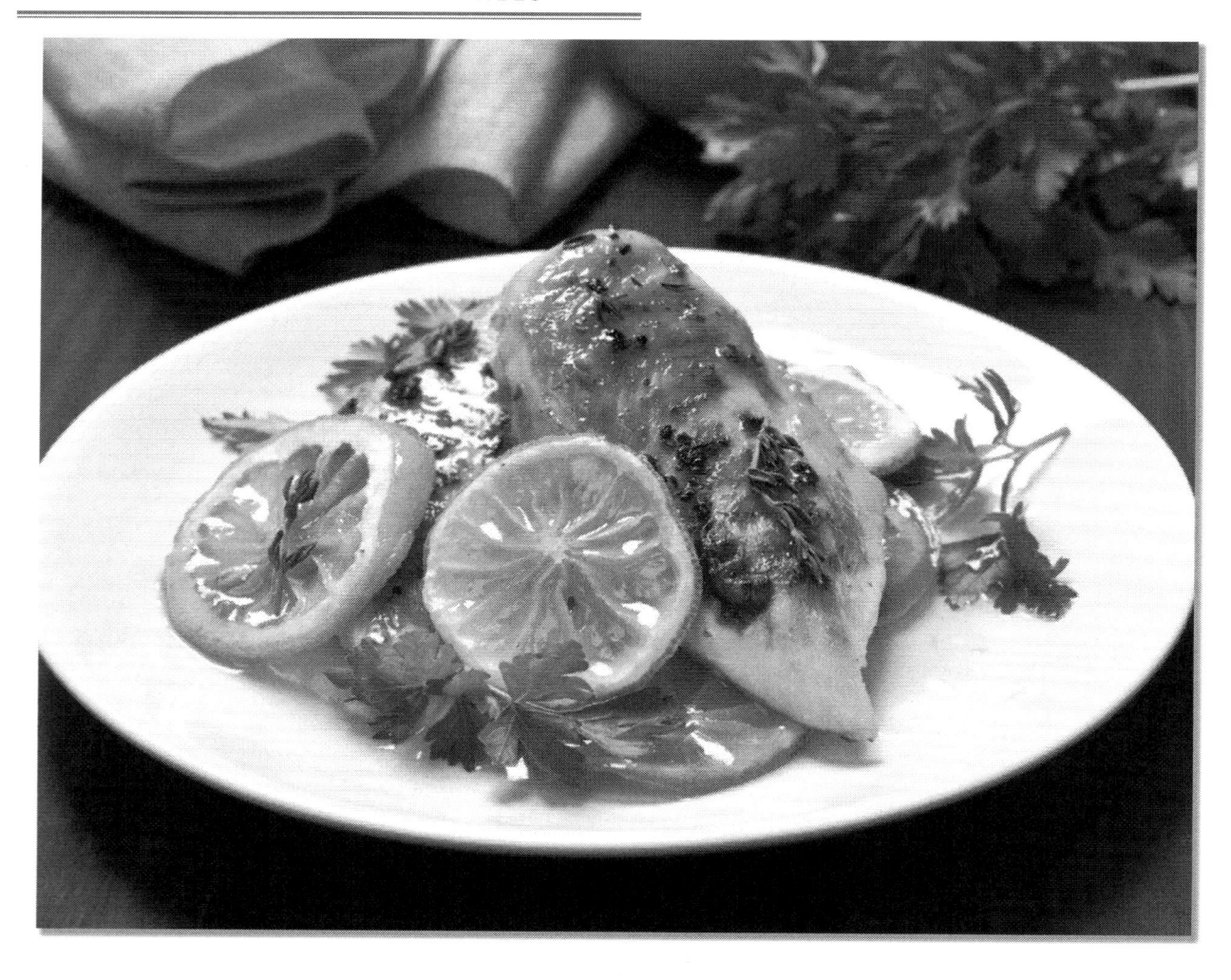

BAKED PORK CHOPS

PREPARATION: 15 min.
COOKING TIME: 40 min.
SERVING: 6 People

Ingredients:

- 1/2 cup flour
- 1 large egg
- 1/4 cup water
- 3/4 cup breadcrumbs
- 6 (3 1/2 oz.) pork chops
- 2 tablespoons butter, unsalted
- 1 teaspoon paprika

Direction:

1. Begin by switching the oven to 350 degrees F to preheat.
2. Mix and spread the flour in a shallow plate.
3. Whisk the egg with water in another shallow bowl.
4. Spread the breadcrumbs on a separate plate.
5. Firstly, coat the pork with flour, then dip in the egg mix and then in the crumbs.
6. Grease a baking sheet and place the chops in it.
7. Drizzle the pepper on top and bake for 40 minutes.
8. Serve.

Nutrition: Calories: 221 kcal, Total Fat: 7.8 g, Saturated Fat: 1.9 g, Cholesterol: 93 mg, Sodium: 135 mg, Total Carbs: 11.9 g, Fiber: 3.5 g, Sugar: 0.5 g, Protein: 24.7 g

BEEF KABOBS WITH PEPPER

PREPARATION: 5 min.
COOKING TIME: 10 min.
SERVING: 8 People

Ingredients:

- 1 Pound of beef sirloin
- ½ Cup of vinegar
- 2 tbsp of salad oil
- 1 Medium, chopped onion
- 2 tbsp of chopped fresh parsley
- ¼ tsp of black pepper
- 2 Cut into strips green peppers

Directions:

1. Trim the fat from the meat; then cut it into cubes of 1 and ½ inches each
2. Mix the vinegar, the oil, the onion, the parsley, and the pepper in a bowl
3. Place the meat in the marinade and set it aside for about 2 hours; make sure to stir from time to time.
4. Remove the meat from the marinade and alternate it on skewers instead with green pepper
5. Brush the pepper with the marinade and broil for about 10 minutes 4 inches from the heat
6. Serve and enjoy your kabobs

Nutrition: Calories: 357 kcal, Total Fat: 24 g, Saturated Fat: 0 g, Cholesterol: 9 mg, Sodium: 60 mg, Total Carbs: 0 g, Fiber :23 g, Sugar: 0 g, Protein: 26 g

CABBAGE AND BEEF FRY

PREPARATION: 5 min.
COOKING TIME: 15 min.
SERVING: 4 People

Ingredients:

- 1 pound beef, ground
- ½ pound bacon
- 1 onion
- 1 garlic clove, minced
- ½ head cabbage
- Salt and pepper to taste

Direction:

1. Take a skillet and place it over medium heat
2. Add chopped bacon, beef and onion until slightly browned
3. Transfer to a bowl and keep it covered
4. Add minced garlic and cabbage to the skillet and cook until slightly browned
5. Return the ground beef mixture to the skillet and simmer for 3-5 minutes over low heat
6. Serve and enjoy!

Nutrition: Calories: 360 kcal, Total Fat: 22 g, Cholesterol: 0 mg, Sodium: 0 mg, Total Carbs: 5 g, Fiber:0 g, Sugar: 0 g, Protein: 34 g

MUSHROOM AND OLIVE SIRLOIN STEAK

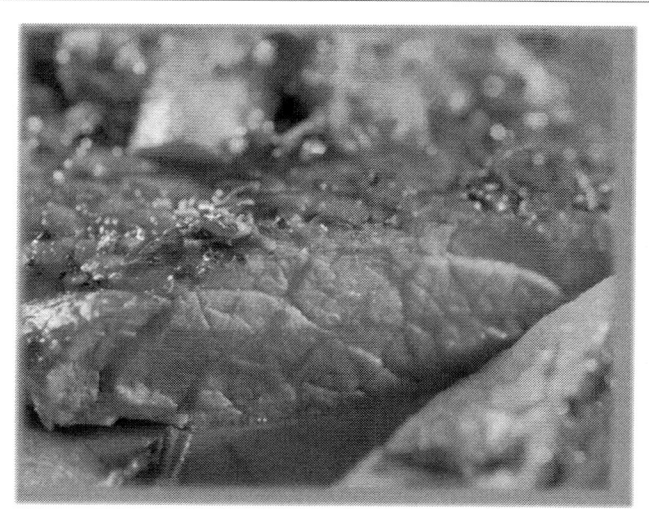

PREPARATION: 10 min.
COOKING TIME: 14 min.
SERVING: 4 People

Ingredients:

- 1-pound boneless beef sirloin steak, ¾ inch thick, cut into 4 pieces
- 1 large red onion, chopped
- 1 cup mushrooms
- 4 garlic cloves, thinly sliced
- 4 tablespoons olive oil
- ½ cup green olives, coarsely chopped
- 1 cup parsley leaves, finely cut

Direction:

1. Take a large-sized skillet and place it over medium-high heat
2. Add oil and let it heat p
3. Add beef and cook until both sides are browned, remove beef and drain fat
4. Add the rest of the oil to skillet and heat it up
5. Add onions, garlic and cook for 2-3 minutes
6. Stir well

7. Add mushrooms olives and cook until mushrooms are thoroughly done
8. Return beef to skillet and lower heat to medium
9. Cook for 3-4 minutes (covered)
10. Stir in parsley
11. Serve and enjoy!

Nutrition: Calories: 386 kcal, Total Fat: 30 g, Saturated Fat: 0 g, Cholesterol: 0 mg, Sodium: 0 mg, Total Carbs: 11 g, Fiber: 0 g, Sugar: 0 g, Protein: 21 g

CALIFORNIA PORK CHOPS

PREPARATION: 10 min.
COOKING TIME: 10 min.
SERVING: 2 People

Ingredients:

- 1 tbsp fresh cilantro, chopped
- 1/2 cup chives, chopped
- 2 large green bell peppers, chopped
- 1 lb. 1" thick boneless pork chops
- 1 tbsp fresh lime juice
- 2 cups cooked rice
- 1/8 tsp dried oregano leaves
- 1/4 tsp ground black pepper
- 1/4 tsp ground cumin
- 1 tbsp butter
- 1 lime

Directions:

1. Start by seasoning the pork chops with lime juice and cilantro.
2. Place them in a shallow dish.
3. Toss the chives with pepper, cumin, butter, oregano and rice in a bowl.
4. Stuff the bell peppers with this mixture and place them around the pork chops.
5. Cover the chop and bell peppers with a foil sheet and bake them for 10 minutes in the oven at 375 degrees f.
6. Serve warm.

Nutrition: Calories: 265 kcal, Total Fat: 15 g, Cholesterol: 86 mg, Sodium: 70 mg, Total Carbs: 24 g, Fiber: 1 g, Sugar: 0 g, Protein: 34 g

BEEF CHORIZO

PREPARATION: 10 min.
COOKING TIME: 10 min.
SERVING: 4 People

Ingredients:

- 3 garlic cloves, minced
- 1 lb. 90% lean ground beef
- 2 tbsp hot chili powder
- 2 tsp red or cayenne pepper
- 1 tsp black pepper
- 1 tsp ground oregano
- 2 tsp white vinegar

Directions:

1. Mix all ingredients together in a bowl thoroughly then spread the mixture in a baking pan.
2. Bake the meat for 10 minutes at 325 degrees f in an oven.
3. Slice and serve in crumbles.

Nutrition: Calories: 72 kcal, Total Fat: 4 g, Saturated Fat: 0 g, Cholesterol: 25 mg, Sodium: 46 mg, Total Carbs: 1 g, Fiber: 0.8 g, Sugar: 0 g, Protein: 8 g

PORK FAJITAS

PREPARATION: 10 min.
COOKING TIME: 20 min.
SERVING: 4 People

Ingredients:

- 1 green bell pepper, julienned
- 1 medium onion, julienned
- 2 garlic cloves, minced
- 1 lb. lean, boneless pork cut into strips
- 1 tsp dried oregano
- 1/2 tsp cumin
- 2 tbsp pineapple juice
- 2 tbsp vinegar
- 1/4 tsp hot pepper sauce
- 1 tbsp canola oil
- 4 flour tortillas, 8" size

Directions:

1. Start by mixing the oregano, garlic, vinegar, cumin, hot sauce, and pineapple juice in a bowl.
2. Place the pork in this marinade and mix well to coat them then refrigerate for 15 minutes.
3. Meanwhile, preheat the oven to 325 degrees f.
4. Wrap the tortillas in a foil and heat them in the oven 2-3 minutes.
5. Now, heat a suitable griddle on medium heat and add pork strips, green peppers, oil, and onion.
6. Cook for 5 minutes until pork is done.
7. Serve warm in warmed tortillas.

Nutrition: Calories: 406 kcal, Total Fat: 18 g, Cholesterol: 64 mg, Sodium: 376 mg, Total Carbs: 34 g, Fiber: 2.4 g, Sugar: 0 g, Protein: 26 g

CARIBBEAN TURKEY CURRY

PREPARATION: 10 min.
COOKING TIME: 1 hour and 30 minutes
SERVING: 6 People

Ingredients:

- 3 1/2 lbs. turkey breast, with skin
- 1/4 cup butter, melted
- 1/4 cup honey
- 1 tbsp mustard
- 2 tsp curry powder
- 1 tsp garlic powder

Directions:

1. Place the turkey breast in a shallow roasting pan.
2. Insert a meat thermometer to monitor the temperature.
3. Bake the turkey for 1.5 hours at 350 degrees f until its internal temperature reaches 170 degrees f.
4. Meanwhile, thoroughly mix honey, butter, curry powder, garlic powder, and mustard in a bowl.
5. Glaze the cooked turkey with this mixture liberally.
6. Let it sit for 15 minutes for absorption.
7. Slice and serve.

Nutrition: Calories: 275 kcal, Total Fat: 13 g, Cholesterol: 82 mg, Sodium: 122 mg, Total Carbs: 90 g, Fiber: 0.2 g, Sugar: 0 g, Protein: 26 g

CHICKEN FAJITAS

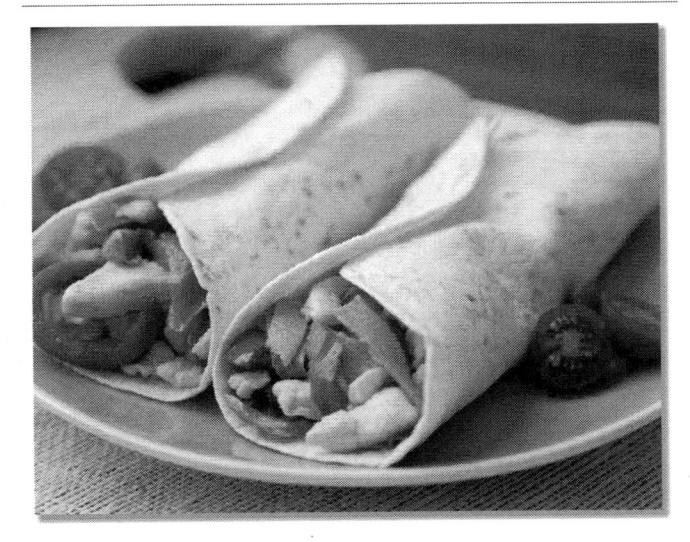

PREPARATION: 10 min.
COOKING TIME: 10 min.
SERVING: 8 People

Ingredients:

- 8 flour tortillas, 6" size
- 1/4 cup green pepper, cut in strips
- 1/4 cup red pepper, cut in strips
- 1/2 cup onion, sliced
- 1/2 cup cilantro
- 2 tbsp canola oil
- 12 oz boneless chicken breasts
- 1/4 tsp black pepper
- 2 tsp chili powder
- 1/2 tsp cumin
- 2 tbsp lemon juice

Directions:

1. Start by wrapping the tortillas in a foil.
2. Warm them up for 10 minutes in a preheated oven at 300 degrees f.
3. Add oil to a nonstick pan.
4. Add lemon juice chicken and seasoning
5. Stir fry for 5 minutes then add onion and peppers.
6. Continue cooking for 5 minutes or until chicken is tender.
7. Stir in cilantro, mix well and serve in tortillas.

Nutrition: Calories: 343 kcal, Total Fat: 13 g, Cholesterol: 53 mg, Sodium: 281 mg, Total Carbs: 33 g, Fiber: 2 g, Sugar: 0 g, Protein: 24 g

CHICKEN VERONIQUE

PREPARATION: 10 min.
COOKING TIME: 10 min.
SERVING: 4 People

Ingredients:

- 2 boneless skinless chicken breasts
- ½ shallot, chopped
- 2 tablespoons butter
- 2 tablespoons dry white wine
- 2 tablespoons chicken broth
- ½ cup green grapes, halved
- 1 teaspoon dried tarragon
- ¼ cup cream

Directions:

1. Place an 8-inch skillet over medium heat and add butter to melt.
2. Sear the chicken in the melted butter until golden-brown on both sides.
3. Place the boneless chicken on a plate and set it aside.
4. Add shallot to the same skillet and stir until soft.
5. Whisk cornstarch with broth and wine in a small bowl.
6. Pour this slurry into the skillet and mix well.
7. Place the chicken in the skillet and cook it on a simmer for 6 minutes.
8. Transfer the chicken to the serving plate.
9. Add cream, tarragon, and grapes.
10. Cook for 1 minute, then pour this sauce over the chicken.
11. Serve.

Nutrition: Calories: 306 kcal, Total Fat: 18 g, Cholesterol: 124 mg, Sodium: 167 mg, Total Carbs: 9 g, Fiber: 0.5 g, Sugar: 0 g, Protein: 27 g

LONDON BROIL

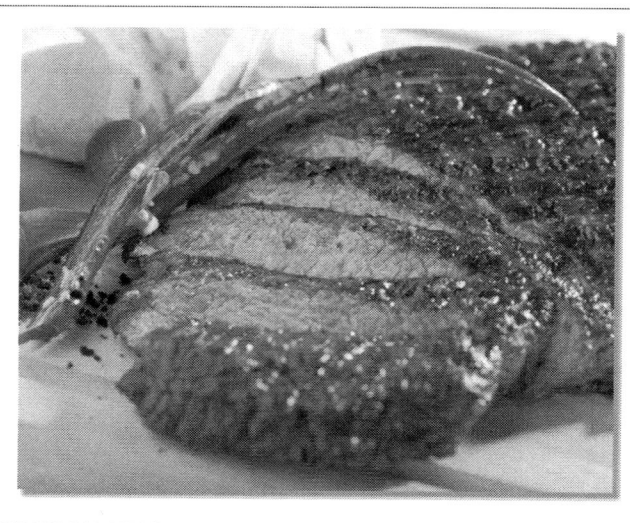

PREPARATION: 10 min.
COOKING TIME: 5 min.
SERVING: 4 People

Ingredients:

- 2 pounds flank steak
- ¼ teaspoon meat tenderizer
- 1 tablespoon sugar
- 2 tablespoons lemon juice
- 2 tablespoons soy sauce
- 1 tablespoon honey
- 1 teaspoon herb seasoning blend

Directions:

1. Pound the meat with a mallet then place it in a shallow dish.
2. Sprinkle meat tenderizer over the meat.
3. Whisk rest of the ingredients and spread this marinade over the meat.
4. Marinate the meat for 4 hours in the refrigerator.
5. Bake the meat for 5 minutes per side at 350ºF.
6. Slice and serve.

Nutrition: Calories: 184 kcal, Total Fat: 8 g, Saturated Fat: 0 g, Cholesterol: 43 mg, Sodium: 208 mg, Total Carbs: 3 g, Fiber: 0 g, Sugar: 0 g, Protein: 24 g

SIRLOIN WITH SQUASH AND PINEAPPLE

PREPARATION: 10 min.
COOKING TIME: 9 min.
SERVING: 2 People

Ingredients:
- 8 ounces canned pineapple slices
- 2 garlic cloves, minced
- 2 teaspoons ginger root, minced
- 3 teaspoons olive oil
- 1 pound sirloin tips
- 1 medium zucchini, diced
- 1 medium yellow squash, diced
- ½ medium red onion, diced

Directions:
1. Mix pineapple juice with 1 teaspoon olive oil, ginger, and garlic in a Ziplock bag.
2. Add sirloin tips to the pineapple juice marinade and seal the bag.
3. Place the bag in the refrigerator overnight.
4. Preheat oven to 450ºF.
5. Layer 2 sheet pans with foil and grease it with 1 teaspoon olive oil.
6. Spread the squash, onion, and pineapple rings in the prepared pans.
7. Bake them for 5 minutes then transfer to the serving plate.
8. Place the marinated sirloin tips on a baking sheet and bake for 4 minutes in the oven.
9. Transfer the sirloin tips to the roasted vegetables.
10. Serve.

Nutrition: Calories: 264 kcal Total Fat: 12 g Cholesterol: 74 mg Sodium: 150 mg Total Carbs: 14 g Fiber: 1.3 g Sugar: 0 g Protein: 25 g

SLOW-COOKED BBQ BEEF

PREPARATION: 10 min.
COOKING TIME: 30 min.
SERVING: 4 People

Ingredients:
- 4-pound pot roast
- 2 cups of water
- ¾ cup ketchup
- ¼ cup brown sugar
- 1/3 cup vinegar
- ½ teaspoon allspice
- ¼ cup onion

Directions:
1. Add 2 cups water and roast to a Crockpot and cover it.
2. Cook for 10 hours on LOW setting, then drain it while keeping 1 cup of its liquid.
3. Transfer the cooked meat to a 9x13 pan and set it aside.
4. Whisk 1 cup liquid, ketchup, vinegar, brown sugar, minced onion, and allspice in a bowl.
5. Add beef to the marinade and mix well to coat, then marinate overnight in the refrigerator.
6. Spread it on a baking pan then bake for 30 minutes at 350ºF.
7. Serve.

Nutrition: Calories: 303 kcal, Total Fat: 17 g, Cholesterol: 71 mg, Sodium: 207 mg, Total Carbs: 7 g, Fiber: 0.2 g, Sugar: 0 g, Protein: 27 g

BARLEY CHICKEN SALAD

PREPARATION: 20 min.
COOKING TIME: 6 min.
SERVING: 6 People

Ingredients:

- ¾ cup quick-cooking barley
- 2½ cups low-sodium chicken broth
- 5 tablespoons olive oil, divided
- 12 ounces boneless skinless chicken breasts, cubed
- Juice of 1 lemon
- 1 tablespoon yellow mustard
- ½ teaspoon dried oregano leaves
- 1 cucumber, peeled and sliced
- 1 red bell pepper, chopped
- 1 cup frozen corn, thawed and drained

Directions:

1. In a medium saucepan over high heat, combine the barley and chicken broth and bring to a simmer.
2. Reduce the heat to low, partially cover the pan, and simmer for 10 to 12 minutes or until the barley is tender.
3. While the barley is cooking, heat 2 tablespoons olive oil in a medium skillet over medium heat.
4. Add the chicken and cook, stirring occasionally, until the chicken is fully cooked to 165°F internal temperature, 5 to 6 minutes. Remove the skillet from the heat.
5. In a serving bowl, whisk the remaining 3 tablespoons olive oil, lemon juice, mustard, and oregano until blended.
6. Add the cooked chicken, barley, cucumber, bell pepper, and corn and toss to coat.
7. This salad can be served warm or chilled in the refrigerator for 2 hours first.

Nutrients: Calories: 281, Potassium: 475mg, Phosphorous: 220mg, Protein: 18g, Sodium: 87mg, Fat: 2g

CHICKEN COLESLAW SALAD

PREPARATION: 10 min.
COOKING TIME: 10 min.
SERVING: 2 People

Ingredients:

- 2 tablespoons olive oil
- 12 ounces boneless skinless chicken breasts, cubed
- Pinch salt
- 1/8 teaspoon freshly ground black pepper
- 1/3 cup mayonnaise
- 2 tablespoons mustard
- Juice of 1 lemon
- 1 teaspoon dried dill weed
- 3 cups chopped red cabbage
- 3 cups chopped green cabbage
- 1½ cups grated carrots

Directions:

1. Heat a medium skillet over medium heat and add the olive oil.
2. Season the chicken with the salt and pepper and add to the skillet. Sauté the chicken. Remove the chicken from the skillet with a slotted spoon to a clean plate and set aside.
3. In a serving bowl, stir together the mayonnaise, mustard, lemon juice, and dill weed until well mixed.
4. Stir in the chicken, red cabbage, green cabbage, and carrots and toss to coat.
5. Serve immediately or cover and chill up to 2 hours before serving.

Nutrition: Calories: 229; Total fat: 15g; Saturated fat: 2g; Sodium: 197mg; Potassium: 463mg; Phosphorus: 162mg; Carbohydrates: 9g; Fiber: 3g; Protein: 14g; Sugar: 4g

BERRY-CHICKEN PASTA SALAD

PREPARATION: 20 min.
COOKING TIME: 6 min.
SERVING: 6 People

Ingredients:

- 8 ounces whole-wheat ziti or penne pasta
- 5 tablespoons olive oil, divided
- 12 ounces boneless skinless chicken breasts, cubed
- Pinch salt
- 1/8 teaspoon freshly ground black pepper
- Juice of 1 lemon
- 2 teaspoons honey
- ½ teaspoon dried thyme leaves
- 2 cups blueberries
- 1 cup sliced strawberries
- 1 cup raspberries

Directions:

1. Bring a large pot of water to a boil. Add the pasta and cook according to package directions until al dente. Drain and set aside.
2. While the pasta is cooking, heat 2 tablespoons of olive oil in a medium skillet over medium heat.
3. Season the chicken with the salt and pepper and add to the skillet. Sauté for 5 to 6 minutes or until the chicken is thoroughly cooked to 165°F internal temperature. Remove the chicken from the skillet with a slotted spoon to a clean plate.
4. In a serving bowl, whisk the remaining 3 tablespoons of olive oil, lemon juice, honey, and thyme leaves until blended.
5. Stir in the cooked pasta, chicken, blueberries, and strawberries until combined.
6. Just before serving, top with the raspberries.

Nutrition: Calories: 357; Total fat: 14g; Saturated fat: 2g; Sodium: 55mg; Potassium: 472mg; Phosphorus: 269mg; Carbohydrates: 42g; Fiber: 7g; Protein: 19g; Sugar: 10g

MEXICAN-STYLE CHICKEN SALAD

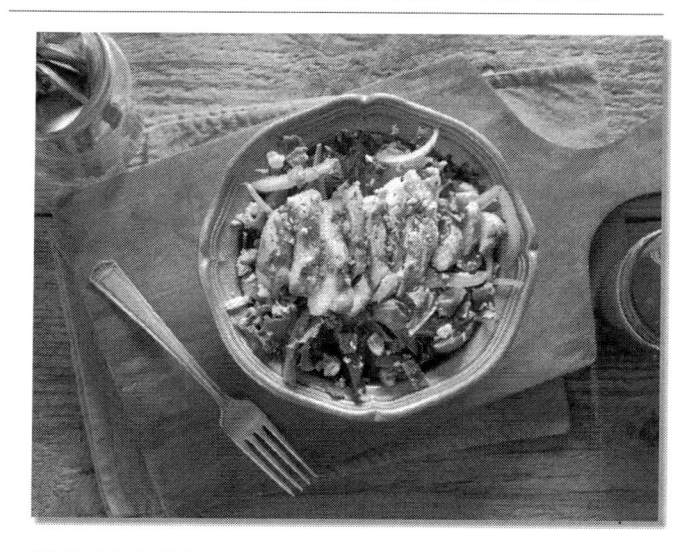

PREPARATION: 20 min.
COOKING TIME: 8 min.
SERVING: 6 People

Ingredients:

- 4 tablespoons olive oil, divided
- 12 ounces boneless skinless chicken thighs, cubed
- 3 teaspoons chili powder, divided
- 1/8 teaspoon cayenne pepper
- 2 tablespoons freshly squeezed lime juice
- 3 cups butter lettuce
- 1 red bell pepper, chopped
- 1½ cups frozen corn, thawed and drained
- 1 jalapeño pepper, minced
- 1 cup crushed yellow tortilla chips
- ½ cup Powerhouse Salsa

Directions:

1. Heat two tablespoons of oil in a medium skillet over medium heat.
2. Sprinkle the chicken thighs with 1 teaspoon chili powder and the cayenne pepper and cook, stirring frequently, for 6 to 8 minutes or until the chicken registers 165°F internal temperature.
3. Transfer the chicken to a serving bowl and add the remaining olive oil, remaining chili powder, and the lime juice. Toss to combine.
4. Add the butter lettuce, bell pepper, corn, and jalapeño pepper and toss.
5. Top with the tortilla chips and the salsa and serve

Nutrition: Calories: 270; Total fat: 15g; Saturated fat: 2g; Sodium: 161mg; Potassium: 489mg; Phosphorus: 186mg; Carbohydrates: 22g; Fiber: 4g; Protein: 14g; Sugar: 4g

SATAY-INSPIRED CHICKEN SALAD

PREPARATION: 20 min.
COOKING TIME: 6 min.
SERVING: 5 People

Ingredients:

- 3 tablespoons olive oil, divided
- 12 ounces boneless skinless chicken breasts, cubed
- 1/8 teaspoon cayenne pepper
- 1/3 cup crunchy peanut butter
- ¼ cup low-sodium chicken broth
- Juice of 1 lemon
- 1/8 teaspoon red pepper flakes
- 1 cup grated carrot
- 3 scallions, white and green parts, sliced
- 2 cups chopped iceberg lettuce
- 2 cups chopped red cabbage

Directions:

1. Heat 2 tablespoons of olive oil in a medium skillet over medium heat.
2. Sprinkle the chicken with cayenne pepper and add to the skillet.

3. Transfer the chicken to a clean plate and set aside.

4. In a medium bowl, whisk the peanut butter, broth, lemon juice, red pepper flakes, and the remaining olive oil until blended.

5. Stir in the chicken, carrot, and scallions until well mixed.

6. Place the lettuce and cabbage into a serving bowl and toss to combine. Top with the chicken mixture, toss it all together, and serve.

Nutrition: Calories: 284; Total fat: 19g; Saturated fat: 3g; Sodium: 135mg; Potassium: 544mg; Phosphorus: 231mg; Carbohydrates: 10g; Fiber: 3g; Protein: 20g; Sugar: 5g

GRILLED CHIMICHURRI CHICKEN KEBABS

PREPARATION: 20 min.
COOKING TIME: 10 min.
SERVING: 4 People

Ingredients:

- 12 ounces boneless skinless chicken breasts, cubed
- Pinch salt
- 1/8 teaspoon freshly ground black pepper
- 1 red bell pepper, cubed
- 1 yellow bell pepper, cubed
- 3 scallions, white and green parts, cut into 1-inch pieces
- ½ cup chopped flat-leaf parsley
- ¼ cup chopped cilantro
- 2 garlic cloves, minced
- 3 tablespoons extra-virgin olive oil, divided
- 1 tablespoon red wine vinegar

Directions:

1. Prepare and preheat the grill to medium coals and set a grill 6 inches from the coals.

2. Sprinkle the chicken breast cubes with salt and pepper.

3. Thread the chicken, red bell pepper, yellow bell pepper, and scallions onto 8-inch metal skewers, alternating pieces of chicken with the veggies. Refrigerate

4. In a small bowl, stir together the parsley, cilantro, garlic, 2 tablespoons olive oil, and the vinegar until well mixed.

5. Brush the kebabs with the remaining 1 tablespoon olive oil and grill, turning once, until the chicken is cooked to 165°F internal temperature and the vegetables are tender, 7 to 9 minutes.

6. Place the kebabs on a serving plate and drizzle with the sauce.

7. Serve.

Nutrition: Calories: 217; Total fat: 13g; Saturated fat: 2g; Sodium: 86mg; Potassium: 479mg; Phosphorus: 206mg; Carbohydrates: 5g; Fiber: 1g; Protein: 20g; Sugar: 3g

ROASTED HERB AND LEMON CHICKEN WITH MASHED SWEET POTATOES

PREPARATION: 10 min.
COOKING TIME: 20 min.
SERVING: 4 People

Ingredients:

- 4 medium sweet potatoes, peeled and quartered
- 4 (4-ounce) boneless skinless chicken thighs
- 1 onion, cut into ½-inch pieces
- 1½ cups frozen green beans
- 3 tablespoons olive oil
- Juice of 1 lemon
- 1 teaspoon dried basil leaves
- ½ teaspoon dried thyme leaves
- ½ teaspoon salt, divided
- ¼ teaspoon freshly ground black pepper, divided
- 1 tablespoon unsalted butter
- ½ teaspoon cinnamon

Directions:

1. Preheat the oven to 450°F.
2. Bring a large pot of water to a boil and boil the sweet potatoes for 10 minutes.
3. Drain the potatoes, add more fresh water to the pot, and boil again until soft, about 10 minutes more.
4. While the sweet potatoes are boiling, pat the chicken dry with paper towels; do not rinse. Cut the chicken into cubes.
5. Arrange the chicken, onion, and green beans on a baking sheet with a lip.
6. Drizzle with the olive oil and lemon juice and sprinkle with the basil, thyme, half the salt, and half the pepper. Toss to coat and rearrange in a single layer.
7. Roast for 15 to 20 minutes or until the chicken registers 165°F internal temperature and the vegetables are tender-crisp.
8. When the sweet potatoes are done, drain and mash them with the butter, cinnamon, and the remaining salt and pepper. Serve with the chicken and vegetables.

Nutrition: Calories: 400; Total fat: 18g; Saturated fat: 5g; Sodium: 485mg; Potassium: 590mg; Phosphorus: 284mg; Carbohydrates: 34g; Fiber: 6g; Protein: 26g; Sugar: 11g

CHICKEN AND BROCCOLI PAN BAKE

PREPARATION: 5 min.
COOKING TIME: 25 min.
SERVING: 4 People

Ingredients:

- 16 ounces boneless skinless chicken breasts, cubed
- 1½ cups frozen broccoli florets
- 2 cups frozen sliced carrots
- 4 tablespoons olive oil
- Juice of 1 lemon
- 1 teaspoon dried oregano leaves

Directions:

1. Preheat the oven to 450°F.
2. Arrange the chicken, broccoli, and carrots on a baking sheet with a lip.
3. Drizzle with the olive oil and lemon juice and sprinkle with the oregano. Toss to coat and arrange everything in a single layer.
4. Roast for 15 to 20 minutes until the chicken registers 165°F internal temperature and the vegetables are tender-crisp.
5. Serve.

Nutrition: Calories: 282; Total fat: 17g; Saturated fat: 3g; Sodium: 85mg; Potassium: 578mg; Phosphorus: 276mg; Carbohydrates: 6g; Fiber: 2g; Protein: 27g; Sugar: 2g

MOROCCAN CHICKEN AND VEGETABLE STEW

PREPARATION: 17 min.
COOKING TIME: 13 min.
SERVING: 4 People

Ingredients:

- 2 tablespoons olive oil
- 12 ounces boneless skinless chicken thighs, cubed
- 1 onion, chopped
- 4 garlic cloves, minced
- 2 cups baby carrots
- 1 cup low-sodium chicken broth
- 1 teaspoon ground ginger
- 1 teaspoon ground cumin
- ½ teaspoon paprika
- ½ teaspoon ground turmeric
- Pinch salt
- 1/8 teaspoon freshly ground black pepper
- 1½ cups frozen baby peas

Directions:

1. Heat the olive oil in a large skillet over medium heat.
2. Add the chicken and onion and sauté for 3 minutes or until the chicken begins to brown.
3. Stir in the garlic, carrots, and chicken broth and bring to a simmer.
4. Reduce the heat to low and stir in the ginger, cumin, paprika, turmeric, salt, and pepper. Partially cover and simmer for 6 minutes.
5. Add the peas and simmer for 2 to 4 minutes longer or until the chicken registers 165°F internal temperature and the vegetables are tender-crisp.
6. Serve.

Nutrition: Calories: 295; Total fat: 11g; Saturated fat: 2g; Sodium: 239mg; Potassium: 584mg; Phosphorus: 267mg; Carbohydrates: 18g; Fiber: 5g; Protein: 30g; Sugar: 7g

MUSHROOM TURKEY BURGERS WITH POWERHOUSE SALSA

PREPARATION: 20 min.
COOKING TIME: 10 min.
SERVING: 4 People

Ingredients:

- 1 (8-ounce) package sliced cremini mushrooms
- 2 tablespoons olive oil
- 1 small onion, diced
- ½ pound 93-percent-lean ground turkey
- 1 large egg
- 3 tablespoons crushed puffed rice cereal
- 1 teaspoon dried thyme leaves
- 2 tablespoons unsalted butter
- 4 butter lettuce leaves
- ¼ cup Powerhouse Salsa

Directions:

1. Finely chop the mushrooms in a blender, food processor, or by hand.
2. Heat the olive oil in a large skillet over medium heat. Add the finely chopped mushrooms and onion and sauté, stirring frequently, until the mushrooms have given up their liquid, about 5 to 6 minutes.
3. Remove the mushrooms from the skillet and place in a medium bowl.
4. In another bowl, mix together the ground turkey, egg, crushed puffed rice cereal, and thyme leaves.
5. Mix in the mushroom mixture until well combined and form into 4 patties.
6. Heat the butter in a large skillet over medium heat.
7. Add the turkey patties and cook until they reach 165°F internal temperature, turning once, about 4 minutes per side.
8. Put each patty on a lettuce leaf and top each with 1 tablespoon of the salsa. Serve.

Nutrition: Calories: 285; Total fat: 21g; Saturated fat: 7g; Sodium: 83mg; Potassium: 568mg; Phosphorus: 257mg; Carbohydrates: 7g; Fiber: 1g; Protein: 19g; Sugar: 3g

THAI-STYLE CHICKEN STIR-FRY

PREPARATION: 10 min.
COOKING TIME: 10 min.
SERVING: 4 People

Ingredients:

- ¾ cup low-sodium chicken broth
- 1 tablespoon freshly squeezed lime juice
- 1 tablespoon cornstarch
- 2 teaspoons low-sodium soy sauce
- 1 teaspoon ground ginger
- 1/8 teaspoon red pepper flakes
- 2 tablespoons olive oil
- 12 ounces boneless skinless chicken breasts, cubed
- 2½ cups frozen stir-fry vegetables
- ¼ cup chopped unsalted roasted cashews

Directions:

1. In a small bowl, whisk together the broth, lime juice, cornstarch, soy sauce, ginger, and red pepper flakes. Set aside.
2. Heat the olive oil in a wok or large skillet over medium-high heat.

3. Add the chicken and vegetables and stir-fry for 6 to 8 minutes or until the chicken reaches 165°F internal temperature and the vegetables are hot and tender crisp.
4. Stir in the sauce and stir-fry for 1 to 2 minutes longer or until the sauce thickens and bubbles.
5. Sprinkle with the cashews and serve.

Nutrition: Calories: 309; Total fat: 17g; Saturated fat: 3g; Sodium: 439mg; Potassium: 624mg; Phosphorus: 293mg; Carbohydrates: 16g; Fiber: 3g; Protein: 24g; Sugar: 6g

VEGETABLE AND TURKEY KEBABS

PREPARATION: 20 min.
COOKING TIME: 10 min.
SERVING: 4 People

Ingredients:

- 2 tablespoons olive oil
- 2 tablespoons freshly squeezed lemon juice
- 2 tablespoons yellow mustard
- 1 garlic clove, minced
- 1 teaspoon dried Italian seasoning
- 1 pound turkey tenderloin, cubed
- 16 whole small mushrooms
- 2 red bell peppers, cut into 1-inch pieces

Directions:
1. Prepare and preheat the grill to medium coals and arrange the rack 6 inches from the heat.
2. In a small bowl, whisk together the olive oil, lemon juice, mustard, garlic, and Italian seasoning. Set aside.
3. Thread the turkey, mushrooms, and bell pepper onto 4 (10-inch) metal skewers, alternating meat and vegetables.
4. Place the kebabs on the rack and brush them with some of the olive oil mixture.
5. Close the grill and cook until the turkey reaches 165°F internal temperature, brushing twice with the olive oil mixture and turning the kebabs occasionally.
6. Brush the kebabs with all of the remaining marinade and cook, turning frequently, for 2 minutes longer.
7. Serve.

Nutrition: Calories: 225; Total fat: 9g; Saturated fat: 1g; Sodium: 218mg; Potassium: 557mg; Phosphorus: 288mg; Carbohydrates: 7g; Fiber: 2g; Protein: 29g; Sugar: 4g

TURKEY PHO

PREPARATION: 10 min.
COOKING TIME: 10 min.
SERVING: 2 People

Ingredients:

- 1 tablespoon olive oil
- ½ pound ground white turkey meat
- 2 cups chopped Napa cabbage
- 1 large carrot, peeled and thinly sliced
- 3 scallions, white and green parts, chopped
- 2 garlic cloves, minced
- 1 teaspoon ground ginger
- ¼ teaspoon ground cloves
- 5 cups water
- 4 ounces dry rice noodles
- 1 tablespoon freshly squeezed lime juice

Directions:

1. In a large pot, heat the oil over medium heat.
2. Add the ground turkey, cabbage, carrots, scallions, and garlic. Sauté for 4 to 5 minutes or until the turkey is browned.
3. Add the ginger, cloves, and water and bring to a simmer.
4. Reduce the heat to low and simmer 5 minutes.
5. Stir in the rice noodles and remove the pot from the heat; cover and let stand for 10 minutes or until the noodles are soft.
6. Stir in the lime juice and serve immediately.

Nutrition: Calories: 282; Total fat: 10g; Saturated fat: 2g; Sodium: 126mg; Potassium: 355mg; Phosphorus: 215mg; Carbohydrates: 29g; Fiber: 2g; Protein: 18g; Sugar: 3g

TURKEY-ASPARAGUS RISOTTO

PREPARATION: 10 min.
COOKING TIME: 10 min.
SERVING: 6 People

Ingredients:

- 4 cups low-sodium chicken broth
- 2 tablespoons olive oil
- 1 onion, chopped
- 2 garlic cloves, minced
- 1 pound turkey tenderloin, cubed
- 1½ cups arborio rice or long-grain white rice
- 2 cups asparagus pieces
- 2 tablespoons unsalted butter
- 2 tablespoons grated Parmesan cheese

Directions:

1. In a small saucepan over low heat, pour the broth and bring to a simmer.
2. Heat the oil in a large saucepan over medium heat.
3. Sauté the onion and garlic for 2 minutes.
4. Add the turkey and rice and sauté 2 more minutes.
5. Start adding the broth to the rice mixture, about ½ cup at a time, stirring constantly.
6. When the broth is absorbed, add more broth. You can stir less often as the rice begins to cook, but keep an eye on the pan.
7. After 15 minutes, add the asparagus to the rice mixture. Continue cooking and adding more broth.
8. The risotto is done when the rice is tender, and most of the broth is absorbed. This whole process should take about 20 minutes. You may not need all of the broth. This dish can be soupier or thicker, depending on how much broth you add and your taste.
9. Stir in the butter and cheese and serve immediately.

Nutrition: Calories: 380; Total fat: 11g; Saturated fat: 4g; Sodium: 175mg; Potassium: 498mg; Phosphorus: 297mg; Carbohydrates: 43g; Fiber: 2g; Protein: 26g; Sugar: 2g

TURKEY TENDERLOIN WITH BERRY SAUCE

PREPARATION: 10 min.
COOKING TIME: 12 min.
SERVING: 4 People

Ingredients:

- 2 tablespoons olive oil
- 1 pound turkey tenderloin, cut into 1-inch-thick slices
- 2 tablespoons all-purpose flour
- Pinch salt
- 1/8 teaspoon freshly ground black pepper
- 1 cup sliced strawberries
- 1 cup raspberries
- 2 tablespoons strawberry jam
- Juice from 1 lemon
- 2 tablespoons water

Directions:

1. Heat the olive oil in a large skillet over medium heat.
2. Sprinkle the turkey slices with the flour, salt, and pepper.
3. Add the turkey to the skillet, cut-side down, and cook for 2 to 5 minutes per side, turning once, until it is lightly brown and registers 165°F internal temperature on a meat thermometer. "Cut-side down" means you put the side that touched the knife down in the pan. If you add the turkey to the skillet on the rounded side, it won't brown as well.
4. Transfer the turkey from the skillet to a clean plate and cover with foil to keep warm.
5. Add the strawberries, raspberries, jam, lemon juice, and water to the skillet. Mash the fruit with a potato masher.
6. Simmer the fruit mixture for 2 minutes.
7. Return the turkey to the skillet, stirring to coat with the berry sauce. Heat for 1 minute, then serve.

Nutrition: Calories: 261 Total fat: 9g; Saturated fat: 1g; Sodium: 171mg; Potassium: 403mg; Phosphorus: 252mg; Carbohydrates: 17g; Fiber: 3g; Protein: 28g; Sugar: 8g

DESSERTS

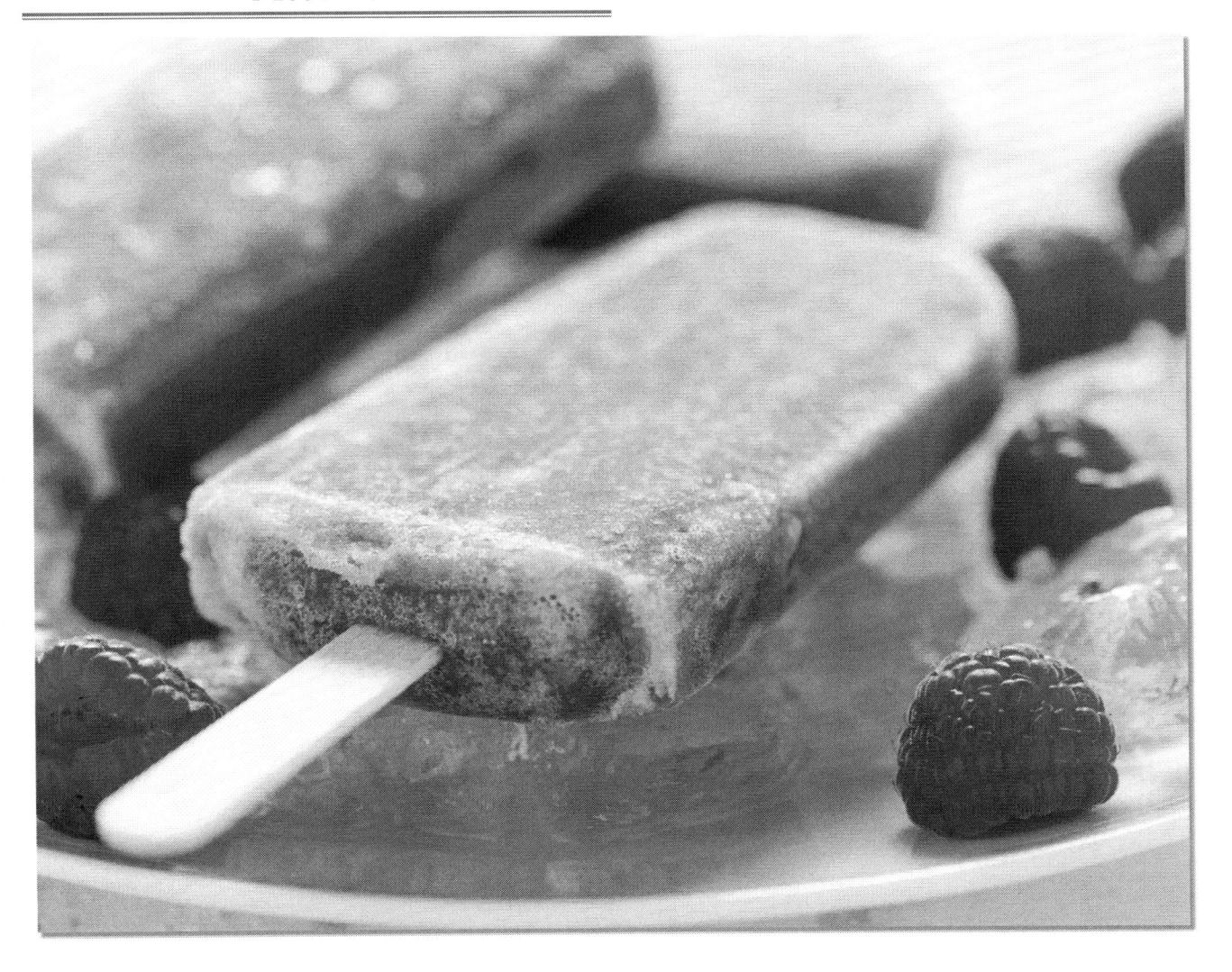

DESSERT COCKTAIL

PREPARATION: 1 min.
COOKING TIME: -
SERVING: 4 People

Ingredients:

- 1 cup of cranberry juice
- 1 cup of fresh ripe strawberries, washed and hull removed
- 2 tablespoon of lime juice
- ¼ cup of white sugar
- 8 ice cubes

Directions:

1. Combine all the ingredients in a blender until smooth and creamy.
2. Pour the liquid into chilled tall glasses and serve cold.

Nutrition: Calories: 92 kcal, Carbohydrate: 23.5 g, Protein: 0.5 g, Sodium: 3.62 mg, Potassium: 103.78 mg, Phosphorus: 17.86 mg, Dietary Fiber: 0.84 g, Fat: 0.17 g

BAKED EGG CUSTARD

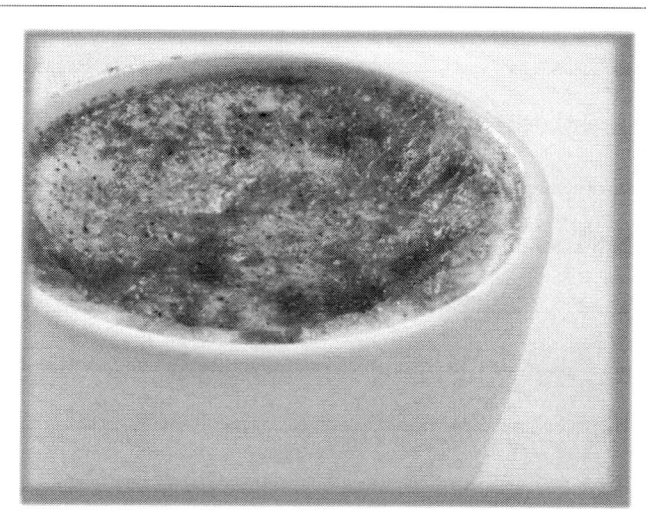

PREPARATION: 10 min.
COOKING TIME: 10 min.
SERVING: 2 People

Ingredients:

- 2 medium eggs, at room temperature
- ¼ cup of semi-skimmed milk
- 3 tablespoons of white sugar
- ½ teaspoon of nutmeg
- 1 teaspoon of vanilla extract

Directions:

1. Preheat your oven at 375 F/180C
2. Mix all the ingredients in a mixing bowl and beat with a hand mixer for a few seconds until creamy and uniform.
3. Pour the mixture into lightly greased muffin tins.
4. Bake for 25-30 minutes or until the knife, you place inside, comes out clean.

Nutrition: Calories: 96.56 kcal, Carbohydrate: 10.5 g, Protein: 3.5 g, Sodium: 37.75 mg, Potassium: 58.19 mg, Phosphorus: 58.76 mg, Dietary Fiber: 0.06 g, Fat: 2.91 g

GUMDROP COOKIES

PREPARATION: 15 min.
COOKING TIME: 12 min.
SERVING: 25 People

Ingredients:

- ½ cup of spreadable unsalted butter
- 1 medium egg
- 1 cup of brown sugar
- 1 2/3 cups of all-purpose flour, sifted
- 1/4 cup of milk
- 1 teaspoon vanilla
- 1 teaspoon of baking powder
- 15 large gumdrops, chopped finely

Directions:

1. Preheat the oven at 400F/195C.
2. Combine the sugar, butter and egg until creamy.
3. Add the milk and vanilla and stir well.
4. Combine the flour with the baking powder in a different bowl. Incorporate to the sugar, butter mixture, and stir.
5. Add the gumdrops and place the mixture in the fridge for half an hour.
6. Drop the dough with tablespoonful into a lightly greased baking or cookie sheet.
7. Bake for 10-12 minutes or until golden brown in color.

Nutrition: Calories: 102.17, kcal Carbohydrate: 16.5 g, Protein: 0.86 g, Sodium: 23.42 mg, Potassium: 45 mg, Phosphorus: 32.15 mg, Dietary Fiber: 0.13 g, Fat: 4 g

APPLE CRUNCH PIE

PREPARATION: 10 min.
COOKING TIME: 35 min.
SERVING: 8 People

Ingredients:

- 4 large tart apples, peeled, seeded and sliced
- ½ cup of white all-purpose flour
- 1/3 cup margarine
- 1 cup of sugar
- ¾ cup of rolled oat flakes
- ½ teaspoon of ground nutmeg

Directions:

1. Preheat the oven to 375F/180C.
2. Place the apples over a lightly greased square pan (around 7 inches).
3. Mix the rest of the ingredients in a medium bowl with and spread the batter over the apples.
4. Bake for 30-35 minutes or until the top crust has gotten golden brown.
5. Serve hot.

Nutrition: Calories: 261.9, kcal Carbohydrate: 47.2 g, Protein: 1.5 g, Sodium: 81 mg, Potassium: 123.74 mg, Phosphorus: 35.27 mg, Dietary Fiber: 2.81 g, Fat: 7.99 g

SPICED PEACHES

PREPARATION: 5 min.
COOKING TIME: 10 min.
SERVING: 2 People

Ingredients:

- Canned peaches with juices – 1 cup
- Cornstarch – ½ teaspoon
- Ground cloves – 1 teaspoon
- Ground cinnamon – 1 teaspoon
- Ground nutmeg – 1 teaspoon
- Zest of ½ lemon
- Water – ½ cup

Directions:

1. Drain peaches.
2. Combine cinnamon, cornstarch, nutmeg, ground cloves, and lemon zest in a pan on the stove.
3. Heat on a medium heat and add peaches.
4. Bring to a boil, reduce the heat and simmer for 10 minutes.
5. Serve.

Nutrition: Calories: 70 Fat: 0g, Carb: 14g, Phosphorus: 23mg, Potassium: 176mg, Sodium: 3mg, Protein: 1g

VANILLA CUSTARD

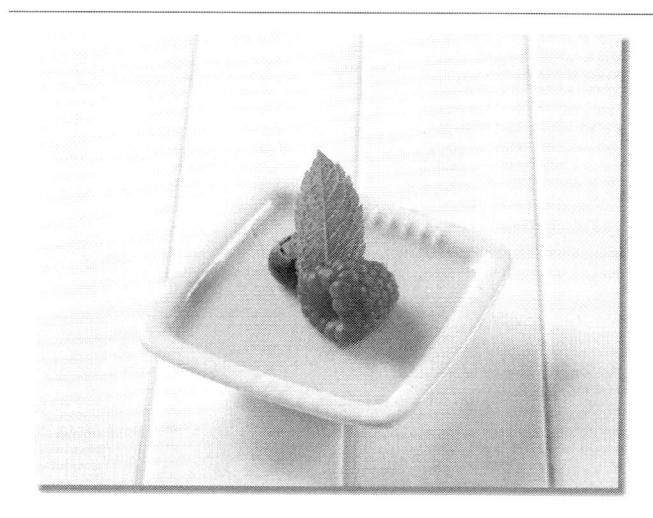

PREPARATION: 7 min.
COOKING TIME: 10 min.
SERVING: 10 People

Ingredients:

- Egg – 1
- Vanilla – 1/8 teaspoon
- Nutmeg – 1/8 teaspoon
- Almond milk – ½ cup
- Stevia - 2 Tablespoon

Directions:

1. Scald the milk then let it cool slightly.
2. Break the egg into a bowl and beat it with the nutmeg.
3. Add the scalded milk, the vanilla, and the sweetener to taste. Mix well.
4. Place the bowl in a baking pan filled with ½ deep of water.
5. Bake for 30 minutes at 325F.
6. Serve.

Nutrition: Calories: 167.3, Fat: 9g, Carb: 11g, Phosphorus: 205mg, Potassium: 249mg, Sodium: 124mg, Protein: 10g

BLUEBERRY AND APPLE CRISP

PREPARATION: 10 min.
COOKING TIME: 25 min.
SERVING: 8 People

Ingredients:

- 4 tbsp cornstarch
- ½ cup brown sugar
- 2 cups grated or chopped apples
- 4 cups of fresh or frozen blueberries (not thawed)
- 1 tbsp lemon juice
- 1 tbsp margarine, melted
- ¼ cup brown sugar
- 1¼ cups quick-cooking rolled oats
- 6 tbsp non-hydrogenated margarine, melted
- ¼ cup unbleached all-purpose flour

Directions:

1. Preheat the oven to 350°F.
2. Combine the dry ingredients in the bowl.
3. Add butter. Stir until moistened. Set aside.
4. Combine cornstarch and brown sugar.
5. Add lemon juice and fruits. Toss.
6. Top with crisp mixture.
7. Bake for 1 hour until golden brown.
8. Serve warm or cold.

Nutrition: Calories: 318.2, Fat: 12g, Protein: 3.3g, Carbohydrates: 52g

LEMON MOUSSE

PREPARATION: 10 min. + chill time
COOKING TIME: 10 min.
SERVING: 4 People

Ingredients:

- 1 cup coconut cream
- 8 ounces cream cheese, soft
- ¼ cup fresh lemon juice
- 3 pinches salt
- 1 teaspoon lemon liquid stevia

Directions:

1. Preheat your oven to 350 °F
2. Grease a ramekin with butter
3. Beat cream, cream cheese, fresh lemon juice, salt and lemon liquid stevia in a mixer
4. Pour batter into ramekin
5. Bake for 10 minutes, then transfer the mousse to a serving glass
6. Let it chill for 2 hours and serve
7. Enjoy!

Nutrition: Calories: 395, Fat: 31g, Carbohydrates: 3g, Protein: 5g

RASPBERRY POPSICLE

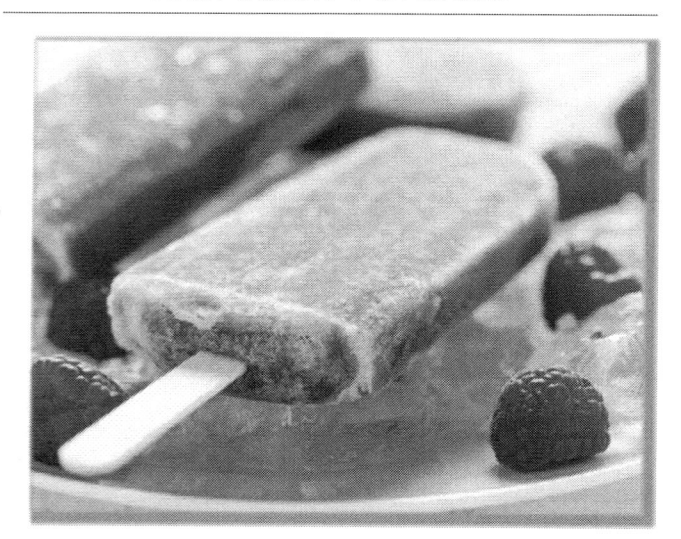

PREPARATION: 2 hours
COOKING TIME: 15 min.
SERVING: 4 People

Ingredients:

- 1 ½ cups raspberries
- 2 cups of water

Directions:

1. Take a pan and fill it up with water
2. Add raspberries
3. Place it over medium heat and bring to water to a boil
4. Reduce the heat and simmer for 15 minutes
5. Remove heat and pour the mix into Popsicle molds
6. Add a popsicle stick and let it chill for 2 hours
7. Serve and enjoy!

Nutrition: Calories: 58, Fat: 0.4g, Carbohydrates: 0g, Protein: 1.4g

EASY FUDGE

PREPARATION: 15 min. + chill time
COOKING TIME: 5 min.
SERVING: 25 People

Ingredients:

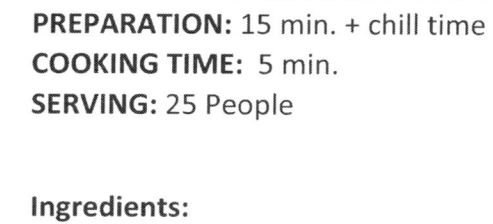

- 1 ¾ cups of coconut butter
- 1 cup pumpkin puree
- 1 teaspoon ground cinnamon
- ¼ teaspoon ground nutmeg
- 1 tablespoon coconut oil

Directions:

1. Take an 8x8 inch square baking pan and line it with aluminum foil
2. Take a spoon and scoop out the coconut butter into a heated pan and allow the butter to melt
3. Keep stirring well and remove from the heat once fully melted
4. Add spices and pumpkin and keep straining until you have a grain-like texture
5. Add coconut oil and keep stirring to incorporate everything
6. Scoop the mixture into your baking pan and evenly distribute it
7. Place wax paper on top of the mixture and press gently to straighten the top
8. Remove the paper and discard
9. Allow it to chill for 1-2 hours
10. Once chilled, take it out and slice it up into pieces
11. Enjoy!

Nutrition: Calories: 120, Fat: 10g, Carbohydrates: 5g, Protein: 1.2g

HEARTY CUCUMBER BITES

PREPARATION: 5 min.
COOKING TIME: -
SERVING: 4 People

Ingredients:

- 1 (8 ounces) cream cheese container, low fat
- 1 tablespoon bell pepper, diced
- 1 tablespoon shallots, diced
- 1 tablespoon parsley, chopped
- 2 cucumbers
- Pepper to taste

Directions:

1. Take a bowl and add cream cheese, onion, pepper, parsley
2. Peel cucumbers and cut in half
3. Remove seeds and stuff with the cheese mix
4. Cut into bite-sized portions and enjoy!

Nutrition: Calories: 85, Fat: 4g, Carbohydrates: 2g, Protein: 3g

CAULIFLOWER BAGEL

PREPARATION: 10 min.
COOKING TIME: 30 min.
SERVING: 12 People

Ingredients:

- 1 large cauliflower, divided into florets and roughly chopped
- ¼ cup nutritional yeast
- ¼ cup almond flour
- ½ teaspoon garlic powder
- 1 ½ teaspoon fine sea salt
- 2 whole eggs
- 1 tablespoon sesame seeds

Directions:

1. Preheat your oven to 400 °F
2. Line a baking sheet with parchment paper, keep it on the side
3. Blend cauliflower in a food processor and transfer to a bowl
4. Add nutritional yeast, almond flour, garlic powder and salt to a bowl, mix
5. Take another bowl and whisk in eggs, add to cauliflower mix
6. Give the dough a stir
7. Incorporate the mix into the egg mix
8. Make balls from the dough, making a hole using your thumb into each ball
9. Arrange them on your prepped sheet, flattening them into bagel shapes
10. Sprinkle sesame seeds and bake for half an hour
11. Remove the oven and let them cool, enjoy!

Nutrition: Calories: 152, Fat: 10g, Carbohydrates: 4g, Protein: 4g

ALMOND CRACKERS

PREPARATION: 10 min.
COOKING TIME: 20 min.
SERVING: 40 crackers

Ingredients:

- 1 cup almond flour
- ¼ teaspoon baking soda
- ¼ teaspoon salt
- 1/8 teaspoon black pepper
- 3 tablespoons sesame seeds
- 1 egg, beaten
- Salt and pepper to taste

Directions:

1. Preheat your oven to 350 °F
2. Line two baking sheets with parchment paper and keep them on the side
3. Mix the dry ingredients into a large bowl and add egg, mix well and form a dough
4. Divide dough into two balls
5. Roll out the dough. Do this between two pieces of parchment paper.
6. Cut into crackers and transfer them to prep a baking sheet
7. Bake for 15-20 minutes
8. Repeat this process until all the dough has been used up
9. Leave crackers to cool and serve
10. Enjoy!

Nutrition: Calories: 302, Fat: 28g, Carbohydrates: 4g, Protein: 9g

CASHEW AND ALMOND BUTTER

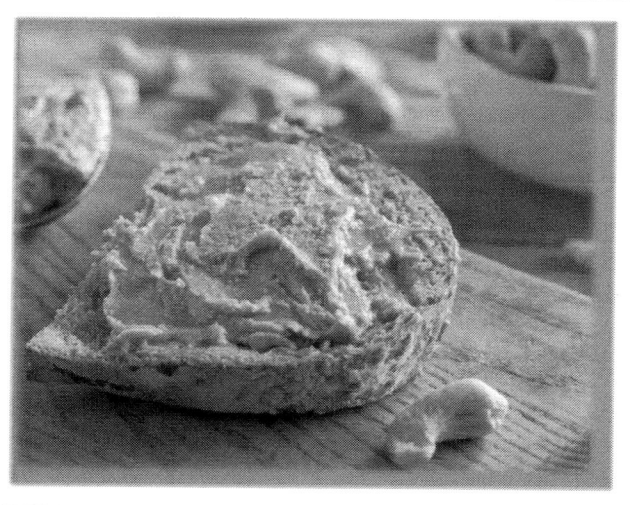

PREPARATION: 5 min.
COOKING TIME: 15 min.
SERVING: 1 ½ cup

Ingredients:

- 1 cup almonds, blanched
- 1/3 cup cashew nuts
- 2 tablespoons coconut oil
- Salt as needed
- ½ teaspoon cinnamon

Directions:

1. Preheat your oven to 350 °F
2. Bake almonds and cashews for 12 minutes
3. Let them cool
4. Transfer to a food processor and add remaining ingredients
5. Add oil and keep blending until smooth
6. Serve and enjoy!

Nutrition: Calories: 205, Fat: 19g, Carbohydrates: 16g Protein: 2.8g

NUT AND CHIA MIX

PREPARATION: 10 min.
COOKING TIME: -
SERVING: 1 person

Ingredients:

- 1 tablespoon chia seeds
- 2 cups of water
- 1-ounce Macadamia nuts
- 1-2 packets Stevia, optional
- 1-ounce hazelnuts

Directions:

1. Add all the listed ingredients to a blender.
2. Blend on high until smooth and creamy.
3. Enjoy your smoothie.

Nutrition: Calories: 452, Fat: 43g, Carbohydrates: 15g, Protein: 9g

VERY BERRY BREAD PUDDING

PREPARATION: 20 min.
COOKING TIME: 60 min.
SERVING: 10 people

Ingredients:

- 8 cups cubed challah bread
- 6 eggs, beaten
- 2 cups heavy cream
- 12-ounce bag of frozen berry medley, thawed
- ½ cup sugar
- 2 teaspoons vanilla
- 1 tablespoon orange zest
- ½ teaspoon cinnamon
- Whipped cream

Directions:

1. Preheat the oven to 375° F.
2. Beat eggs, sugar, cream, orange zest, vanilla and cinnamon until smooth.
3. Mix in bread cubes and fruit with hands.
4. Pour into buttered/greased pan and bake covered in foil for 35 minutes. If using butter, make sure it is unsalted.
5. Remove foil and bake for 15 additional minutes.
6. Turn off oven and let sit in oven for 10 minutes.
7. Cut, then serve topped with whipped cream.

Nutrition: Calories: 392 kcal, Total Fat: 23 g, Cholesterol: 189, mg Sodium: 231 mg, Total Carbs: 36 g, Fiber: 2.2 g, Sugar: 0 g, Protein: 9 g

SUNBURST LEMON BARS

PREPARATION: 10 min.
COOKING TIME: 20 min.
SERVING: 24 people

Ingredients:

Crust:

- 2 cups all-purpose flour
- ½ cup powdered sugar
- 1 cup butter (2 sticks), unsalted, room temperature

Filling:

- 4 eggs
- 1½ cups sugar
- ¼ cup all-purpose flour
- ½ teaspoon cream of tartar
- ¼ teaspoon baking soda
- ¼ cup lemon juice

Glaze:

- 1 cup powdered sugar, sifted
- 2 tablespoons lemon juice

Directions:

Crust:

1. Preheat oven to 350° F.
2. In a large bowl, combine the flour, powdered sugar and 1 cup of softened butter. Mix until crumbly. Press the mixture into the bottom of a 9" x 13" baking pan.
3. Bake until lightly browned, about 15–20 minutes.

Filling:

1. In a medium-sized bowl, whisk the eggs slightly.
2. In another bowl, combine the sugar, flour, cream of tartar and baking soda. Add the dry mixture to the eggs. Add the lemon juice to the egg mixture and whisk until slightly thickened.
3. Pour over the warm crust and bake for another 20 minutes or until filling is set.
4. Remove from the oven and cool.

Glaze:

1. In a small bowl, gradually stir the lemon juice into the sifted powdered sugar until spreadable. Add more or less lemon juice as needed.
2. Spread over the cooled filling. Let the glaze set and then cut into 24 bars. Store extra lemon bars in the refrigerator.

Nutrition: Calories: 200 kcal, Total Fat: 9 g, Saturated Fat: 5 g, Cholesterol: 53 mg, Sodium: 27 mg, Total Carbs: 28g, Fiber: 0.3g, Sugar: 0g, Protein: 2g

CREAMY MINT CHOCOLATE BROWNIES

PREPARATION: 10 min.
COOKING TIME: 20 min.
SERVING: 24 people

Ingredients:

- 1 box Betty Crocker® brownie mix
- 12/14 Andes® mint chocolates
- Optional garnish: fresh mint sprigs, powdered sugar, cocoa powder

Directions:

1. Preheat oven and prepare the brownie mix according to the directions on the box.
2. Prepare 12 cup muffin tin with a liner or lightly grease and flour the bottom and sides.
3. Pour the brownie mix into the pans and bake for 25/27 minutes.
4. Remove brownies from the oven and insert one piece of mint candy in the center and bake for an additional 4/5 minutes.
5. Turn off the oven and remove.
6. Let cool for 5–12 minutes.
7. Remove brownie cupcakes from pan and then serve.

Nutrition: Calories: 308 kcal, Total Fat: 19g, Saturated Fat: 5g, Cholesterol: 33 mg, Sodium: 146 mg, Total Carbs: 37g, Protein: 3g

FESTIVE CREAM CHEESE SUGAR COOKIES

PREPARATION: 5 min.
COOKING TIME: 15 min.
SERVING: 48 people

Ingredients:

- 1 cup sugar
- 1 cup butter, unsalted, softened
- 3 ounces cream cheese, softened
- 1 large egg, separated
- ½ teaspoon salt
- ¼ teaspoon almond extract
- ½ teaspoon vanilla extract
- 2¼ cups all-purpose flour
- Optional garnish: colored sugar

Directions:

1. In a large bowl, combine sugar, butter, cream cheese, salt, almond extract, vanilla extract and egg yolk. Blend well. Stir in flour until well-blended.
2. Chill cookie dough for 2 hours in the refrigerator.
3. Preheat oven to 350° F.
4. On a lightly floured surface, roll out the dough, one third at a time to ¼–inch thickness. Cut into desired shapes with lightly floured cookie cutters.
5. Place them 1 inch apart on ungreased cookie sheets. Leave cookies plain, or if desired, brush with slightly beaten egg white and sprinkle with colored sugar.
6. Bake cream cheese cookies for 7–9 minutes or until light golden brown.
7. Let cool completely before serving.

Nutrition: Calories: 79 kcal, Total Fat: 5g, Saturated Fat: 3g, Cholesterol: 16 mg, Sodium: 33 mg, Total Carbs: 0g, Fiber: 0g, Sugar: 0g, Protein: 1g

DANDELION GREEN SMOOTHIE

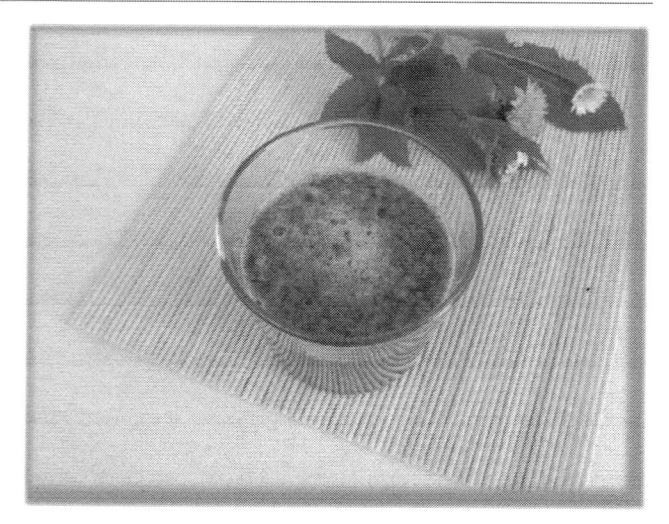

PREPARATION: 20 min.
COOKING TIME: 10 min.
SERVING: 2-4 people

Ingredients:

- 16 - oz filtered water
- 2 - C loosely packed organic dandelion greens, remove the leaves from the stem
- 1 - C organic spinach (loosely packed)
- 1 - organic orange
- 1 - handful of frozen organic strawberries

Directions:

1. Blend all fixings in a blender.
2. Partition into 2 segments and serve

Nutrition: Calories 315g, Fat 8g, Carbs 15g, Sugars 1.2g, Protein 26g

CHOCOLATE CHIP COOKIES

PREPARATION: 7 min.
COOKING TIME: 10 min.
SERVING: 10 people

Ingredients:

- Semi-sweet chocolate chips – ½ cup
- Baking soda – ½ tsp.
- Vanilla – ½ tsp.
- Egg – 1
- Flour – 1 cup
- Margarine – ½ cup
- Stevia – 4 tsp.

Directions:

1. Sift the dry ingredients.
2. Cream the margarine, stevia, vanilla and egg with a whisk.
3. Add flour mixture and beat well.
4. Stir in the chocolate chips, then drop teaspoonfuls of the mixture over a greased baking sheet.
5. Bake the cookies for about 10 minutes at 375F.
6. Cool and serve.

Nutrition: Calories: 106.2 kcal, Total Fat: 7 g, Saturated Fat: 0g, Cholesterol: 0 mg, Sodium: 98 mg, Total Carbs: 8.9g, Fiber: 0 g, Sugar: 0g, Protein: 1.5g

BAKED PEACHES WITH CREAM CHEESE

PREPARATION: 10 min.
COOKING TIME: 15 min.
SERVING: 4 people

Ingredients:

- Plain cream cheese – 1 cup
- Crushed meringue cookies – ½ cup
- Ground cinnamon – ¼ tsp.
- Pinch ground nutmeg
- Canned peach halves – 8, in juice
- Honey – 2 Tbsp.

Directions:

1. Preheat the oven to 350F.
2. Line a baking sheet with parchment paper. Set aside.
3. In a small bowl, stir together the meringue cookies, cream cheese, cinnamon, and nutmeg.
4. Spoon the cream cheese mixture evenly into the cavities in the peach halves.
5. Place the peaches on the baking sheet and bake for 15 minutes or until the fruit is soft and the cheese is melted.
6. Remove the peaches from the baking sheet onto plates.
7. Drizzle with honey and serve.

Nutrition: Calories: 260 kcal, Total Fat: 20 g, Saturated Fat: 0 g, Cholesterol: 0, mg Sodium: 216 mg, Total Carbs: 19g, Fiber: 0g, Sugar: 0g, Protein: 4g

STRAWBERRY ICE CREAM

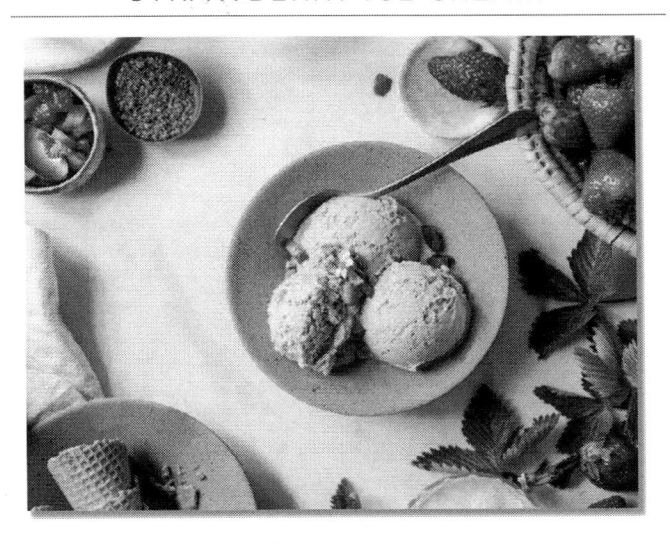

PREPARATION: 5 min.
COOKING TIME: 5 min.
SERVING: 3 people

Ingredients:

- Stevia – ½ cup
- Lemon juice – 1 Tbsp.
- Non-dairy coffee creamer – ¾ cup
- Strawberries – 10 oz.
- Crushed ice – 1 cup

Directions:

1. Blend everything in a blend until smooth.
2. Freeze until frozen.
3. Serve.

Nutrition: Calories: 94.4 kcal, Total Fat: 6g, Saturated Fat: 0g, Cholesterol: 0 mg, Sodium: 25 mg, Total Carbs: 8.3g, Fiber: 0g, Sugar: 0g, Protein: 1.3g

RASPBERRY BRÛLÉE

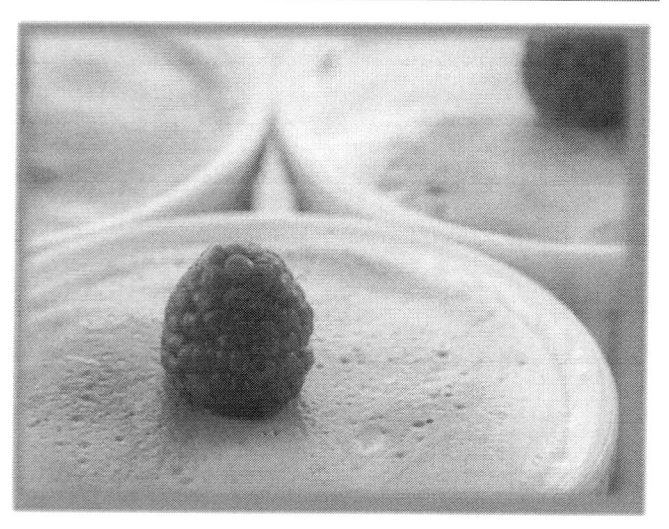

PREPARATION: 5 min.
COOKING TIME: 5 min.
SERVING: 3 people

Ingredients:

- Light sour cream – ½ cup
- Plain cream cheese – ½ cup
- Brown sugar – ¼ cup, divided
- Ground cinnamon – ¼ tsp.
- Fresh raspberries – 1 cup

Directions:

1. Preheat the oven to broil.
2. In a bowl, beat together the cream cheese, sour cream, 2 tbsp. brown sugar and cinnamon for 4 minutes or until the mixture is very smooth and fluffy.
3. Evenly divide the raspberries among 4 (4-ounce) ramekins.
4. Spoon the cream cheese mixture over the berries and smooth the tops.
5. Sprinkle ½ tbsp. brown sugar evenly over each ramekin.
6. Place the ramekins on a baking sheet and broil 4 inches from the heating element until the sugar is caramelized and golden brown.
7. Cool and serve.

Nutrition: Calories: 188 kcal, Total Fat: 13 g, Saturated Fat: 0g, Cholesterol: 0 mg, Sodium: 132 mg ,Total Carbs: 16g, Fiber: 0g, Sugar: 0g, Protein: 3g

SAUCES, DRESSING AND SEASONINGS

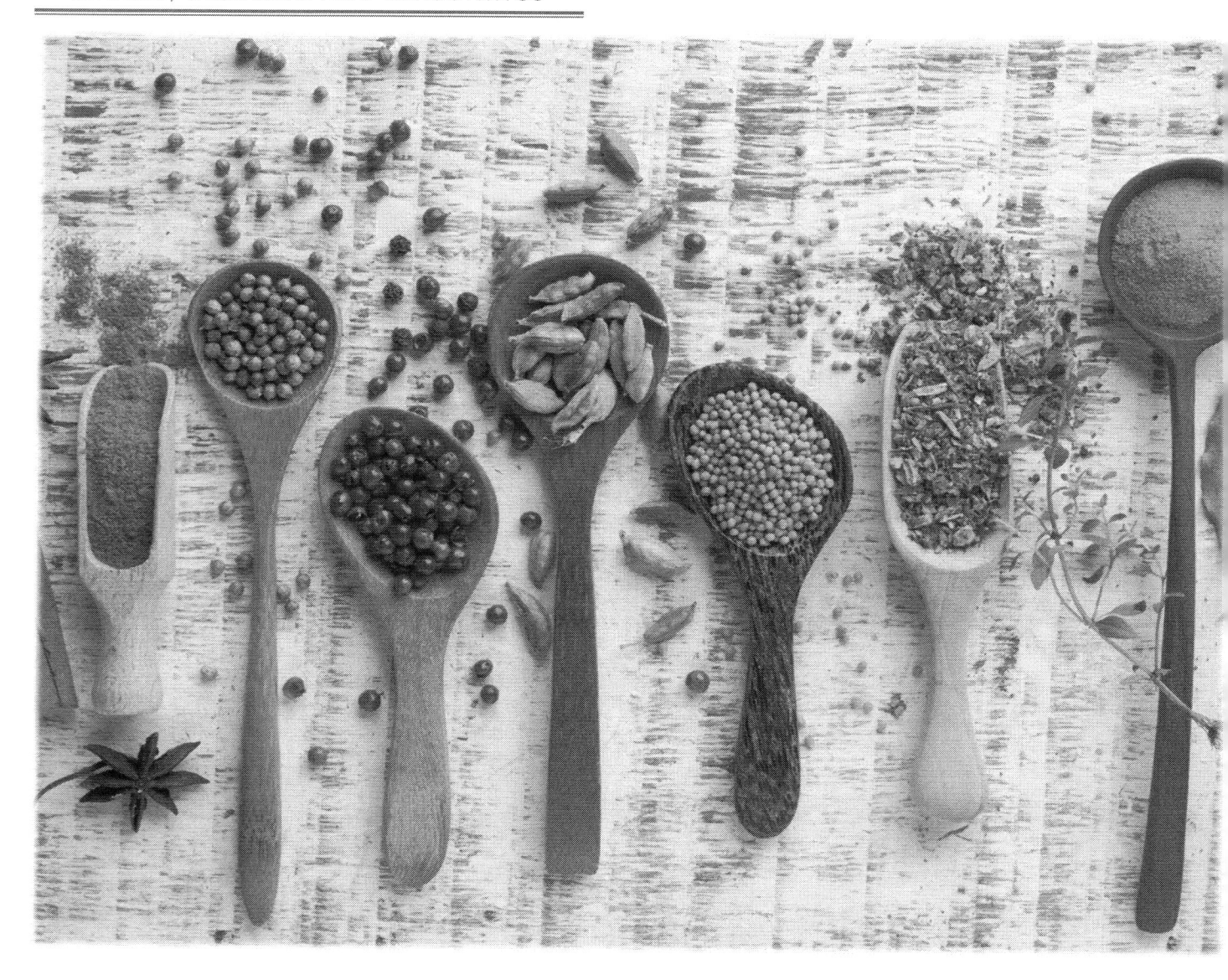

EASY GARLICKY CHERRY TOMATO SAUCE

PREPARATION: 5 min.
COOKING TIME: 25 min.
SERVING: 4 people

Ingredients:

- ¼ cup extra virgin olive oil
- ¼ thinly sliced garlic cloves
- 2 pounds organic cherry tomatoes
- ½ teaspoon dried oregano
- 1 teaspoon coconut sugar
- ¼ cup chopped fresh basil
- 1 teaspoon salt

Directions:

1. Heat oil in a large saucepan over medium heat.
2. Sauté the garlic for a minute until fragrant.
3. Add in the cherry tomatoes and season with salt, oregano, coconut sugar, and fresh basil.
4. Allow to simmer for 25 minutes until the tomatoes are soft and becomes a thick sauce.
5. Place in containers and store in the fridge until ready to use.

Nutrition: Calories 198, Total Fat 6g, Saturated Fat 0.8g, Total Carbs 37g, Net Carbs 32g, Protein 3g, Sugar: 30g, Fiber: 5g, Sodium: 116mg, Potassium 514mg

ROASTED ONION DIP

PREPARATION: 15 min.
COOKING TIME: 35 min.
SERVING: 3 people

Ingredients:

- One red onion, chopped
- Two tablespoons extra-virgin olive oil
- 1 (8-ounce) package cream cheese
- Two tablespoons mayonnaise (made with olive oil)
- One tablespoon freshly squeezed lemon juice
- ½ teaspoon dried thyme leaves

Directions:

1. Preheat the oven to 400°F.
2. On a rimmed baking sheet, combine the onion and olive oil and toss to coat.
3. Roast for 30 to 35 minutes, occasionally stirring, until the onions are soft and golden brown. Don't let them burn. Transfer to a plate and set aside.
4. In a medium bowl, beat the cream cheese, mayonnaise, lemon juice, and thyme leaves. Stir in the onions.
5. You can serve the dip at this point or cover and refrigerate it up to 8 hours before serving.

Nutrition: Calories: 212, Total fat: 21g, Saturated fat: 9g, Sodium: 149mg, Phosphorus: 47mg, Potassium: 82mg, Carbohydrates: 4g, Protein: 3g, Sugar: 2g

GOLDEN TURMERIC SAUCE

PREPARATION: 10 min.
COOKING TIME: 15 min.
SERVING: 4 people

Ingredients:

- 2 tablespoons coconut oil
- 1 onion, chopped
- 2-inch piece ginger, peeled and minced
- 2 cloves of garlic, minced
- 2 cups white sweet potato, cubed
- 2 tablespoons turmeric powder
- ½ teaspoon ginger powder
- ¼ teaspoon cinnamon powder
- 2 cups coconut milk
- Juice from 1 lemon, freshly squeezed
- 1 cup water
- 1 ½ teaspoon salt

Directions:

1. Heat oil in a saucepan over medium flame.
2. Sauté the onion, ginger, and garlic until fragrant.
3. Add in the sweet potatoes, turmeric powder, ginger powder, and cinnamon powder.
4. Pour in water and season with salt.
5. Bring to a boil for 10 minutes.
6. Once the potatoes are soft, place in a blender pulse until smooth.
7. Return the mixture into the saucepan. Turn on the stove.
8. Add in the coconut milk and lemon juice.
9. Allow to simmer for 5 minutes.
10. Store in lidded containers and put inside the fridge until ready to use.

Nutrition: Calories: 172, Total Fat: 11g, Saturated Fat: 2g, Total Carbs: 15g, Net Carbs: 12g, Protein: 5g, Sugar: 8g, Fiber: 3g, Sodium: 36mg, Potassium: 408mg

CREAMY TURMERIC DRESSING

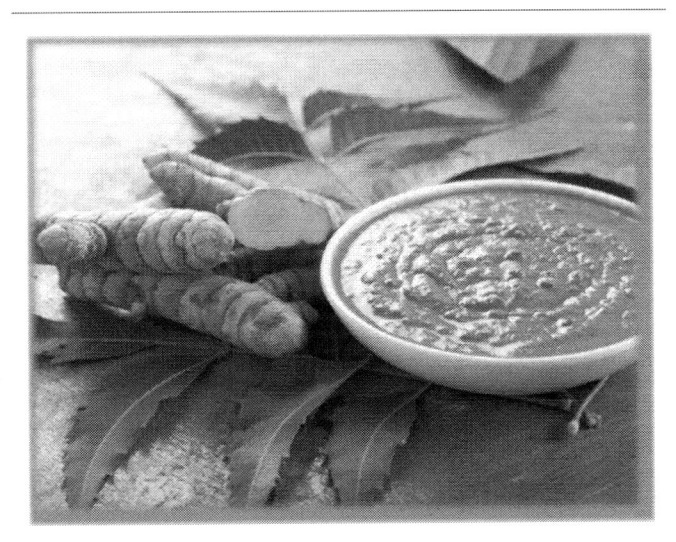

PREPARATION: 5 min.
COOKING TIME: -
SERVING: 6 people

Ingredients:

- ½ cup tahini
- ½ cup olive oil
- 2 tablespoons lemon juice
- 2 teaspoons honey
- Salt to taste
- a dash of black pepper

Directions:

1. Mix all ingredients in a bowl until the mixture becomes creamy and smooth.
2. Store in lidded containers.
3. Put in the fridge until ready to use.

Nutrition: Calories: 286, Total Fat: 29g, Saturated Fat: 4g, Total Carbs: 7g, Net Carbs: 5g, Protein: 4g, Sugar: 2g, Fiber: 2 g, Sodium: 24mg, Potassium: 89mg

DIJON MUSTARD VINAIGRETTE

PREPARATION: 5 min.
COOKING TIME: -
SERVING: 6 people

Ingredients:

- ¾ cup olive oil
- ¼ cup apple cider vinegar
- 3 tablespoons Dijon mustard
- 2 shallots, quartered
- 1 garlic clove, chopped
- A handful of parsley, chopped

Directions:

1. Place all ingredients in a food processor.
2. Pulse until smooth.
3. Place in containers and store in the fridge until ready to use.

Nutrition: Calories: 252, Total Fat: 27g, Saturated Fat: 4g, Total Carbs: 2g, Net Carbs: 1.3g, Protein: 0.6g, Sugar: 1g, Fiber: 0.7g, Sodium: 80 mg, Potassium: 93mg

ANTI-INFLAMMATORY CAESAR DRESSING

PREPARATION: 5 min.
COOKING TIME: -
SERVING: 6 people

Ingredients:

- ½ cup cashew nuts, soaked in water then drained
- 1/3 cup fresh lemon juice
- 1 clove of garlic, minced
- 1 tablespoon Dijon mustard
- 1 tablespoon anchovy paste
- 2 tablespoon extra-virgin olive oil
- ½ cup plain Greek yogurt

Directions:

1. Place all ingredients in a food processor.
2. Pulse until a smooth paste is formed.
3. Place in containers and store in the fridge until ready to use.

Nutrition: Calories: 96, Total Fat: 7g, Saturated Fat: 1.2g, Total Carbs: 5g, Net Carbs: 4.5g, Protein: 4g, Sugar: 1g, Fiber: 0.5g, Sodium: 113mg, Potassium: 132mg

FRESH TOMATO VINAIGRETTE

PREPARATION: 5 min.
COOKING TIME: 25 min.
SERVING: 4 people

Ingredients:

- 1 fresh tomato, chopped
- ¾ cup olive oil
- ¼ cup apple cider vinegar
- 1 clove of garlic, chopped
- ½ teaspoon dried oregano
- Salt and pepper to taste

Directions:

1. Place all ingredients in a food processor.
2. Pulse until a smooth paste is formed.
3. Place in containers and store in the fridge until ready to use.

Nutrition: Calories: 298, Total Fat: 32g, Saturated Fat: 5g, Total Carbs: 2g, Protein: 0.2g, Sugar: 2g, Fiber: 0.4g, Sodium: 3mg, Potassium: 75mg

GINGER SESAME SAUCE

PREPARATION: 5 min.
COOKING TIME: -
SERVING: 6 people

Ingredients:
- ½ cup olive oil
- ¼ cup sesame oil
- 1/3 cup rice wine vinegar
- 1 tablespoon fresh ginger
- 1 tablespoon sesame seeds

Directions:
1. Place all ingredients in a food processor.
2. Pulse until a smooth paste is formed.
3. Place in containers and store in the fridge until ready to use.

Nutrition: Calories: 250, Total Fat: 28g, Saturated Fat: 4g, Total Carbs: 0.2g, Net Carbs: 0.1g, Protein: 0.3g, Sugar: 0.01g, Fiber: 0.1g, Sodium: 2mg, Potassium: 10 mg

GOLDEN TURMERIC TAHINI SAUCE

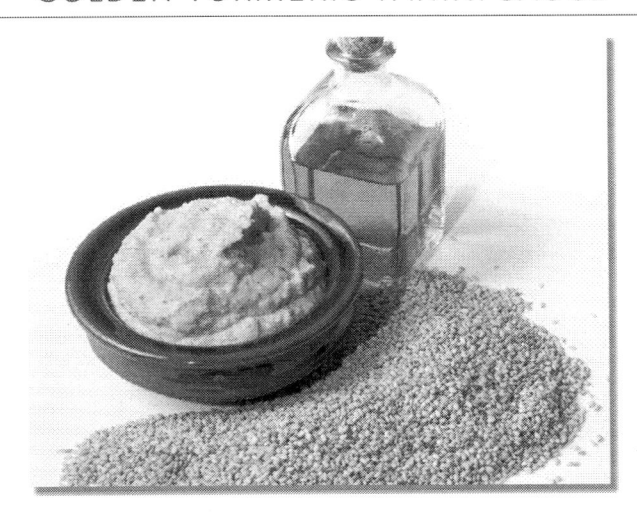

PREPARATION: 5 min.
COOKING TIME: -
SERVING: 6 people

Ingredients:
- ¼ cup tahini
- ¼ cup lemon juice
- 1 tablespoon olive oil
- 1 tablespoon nutritional yeast
- ½ tablespoon maple syrup
- ¼ teaspoon ground turmeric
- A pinch of cayenne pepper
- 2 tablespoons water
- ¼ teaspoon salt
- ¼ teaspoon black pepper

Directions:
1. Place all ingredients in a food processor.
2. Pulse until a smooth paste is formed.
3. Place in containers and store in the fridge until ready to use.

Nutrition: Calories: 71, Total Fat: 6g, Saturated Fat: 1g, Total Carbs: 4 g, Net Carbs: 3g, Protein: 2g, Sugar: 1g, Fiber: 1g, Sodium: 56mg, Potassium: 341mg

HEALTHY TERIYAKI SAUCE

PREPARATION: 5 min.
COOKING TIME: 8 min.
SERVING: 6 people

Ingredients:

- ½ cup reduced-sodium tamari
- ¼ cup pitted dates, pulsed until smooth
- 1 ½ teaspoons minced garlic
- 1 ½ teaspoons minced ginger
- 1 tablespoon blackstrap molasses
- 2 tablespoons sweet rice cooking wine
- 2 teaspoons arrowroot powder + 2 teaspoons water
- ¼ cup water

Directions:

1. Place all ingredients except for the arrowroot slurry in a saucepan.
2. Turn on the heat and bring to a simmer for 5 minutes over medium flame.
3. Add in the arrowroot slurry and continue cooking for another 3 minutes or until the sauce thickens.
4. Place in containers and store in the fridge.

Nutrition: Calorie: 236, Total Fat: 11g, Saturated Fat: 2g, Total Carbs: 31g, Net Carbs: 29g, Protein: 7g, Sugar: 11g, Fiber: 2g, Sodium: 245mg, Potassium: 274mg

YOGURT GARLIC SAUCE

PREPARATION: 5 min.
COOKING TIME: -
SERVING: 4 people

Ingredients:

- 1 cup yogurt
- 1 clove of garlic, minced
- 1/3 cup parsley, finely chopped
- Juice from ½ lemon

Directions:

1. Place all ingredients in a bowl.
2. Whisk to combine everything.
3. Put in a container with lid and store in the fridge until ready to use.

Nutrition: Calories: 42, Total Fat: 2g, Saturated Fat: 1g, Total Carbs: 4g, Net Carbs: 3.8g, Protein: 2g, Sugar: 3g, Fiber:0.2 g, Sodium: 31mg, Potassium: 132mg

CHUNKY TOMATO SAUCE

PREPARATION: 5 min.
COOKING TIME: 15 min.
SERVING: 6 people

Ingredients:

- ¼ cup extra virgin olive oil
- 2 onions, chopped
- 5 cloves of garlic, minced
- 2 red bell peppers, chopped
- ½ cup sliced Portobello mushrooms
- 3 cups diced tomatoes
- 1 teaspoon dried oregano
- 2 teaspoons honey
- 2 teaspoons balsamic vinegar
- 1 teaspoon dried basil
- ½ cup fresh spinach, chopped
- salt and pepper to taste

Directions:

1. In a heavy pan, heat oil over medium flame.
2. Stir in the onions, garlic, and bell pepper until fragrant.
3. Add in the mushrooms, tomatoes, oregano, honey, balsamic vinegar, and basil. Season with salt and pepper to taste.
4. Close the lid and bring to a simmer for 10 minutes until the tomatoes have wilted.
5. Add in the spinach last and cook for another 5 minutes.
6. Place in containers and store in the fridge until ready to use.

Nutrition: Calories: 86, Total Fat: 4g, Saturated Fat: 0.6g, Total Carbs: 11g, Net Carbs: 9g, Protein: 2g, Sugar: 7g, Fiber: 2g, Sodium: 88mg, Potassium: 358mg

SWEET BALSAMIC DRESSING

PREPARATION: 5 min.
COOKING TIME: -
SERVING: 5 people

Ingredients:

- 1 cup olive oil
- ½ cup balsamic vinegar
- 2 teaspoons raw honey
- 2 teaspoons mustard
- 2 cloves of garlic, minced
- Salt and pepper to taste

Directions:

1. Combine all ingredients in a blender and combine until the mixture becomes smooth.
2. Place in contains until ready to use.

Nutrition: Calories: 416, Total Fat: 43g, Saturated Fat: 6g, Total Carbs: 7g, Net Carbs: 6.9g, Protein: 0.3g, Sugar: 6 g, Fiber: 0.1g, Sodium: 29mg, Potassium: 38mg

CITRUS SALAD SAUCE

PREPARATION: 5 min.
COOKING TIME: -
SERVING: 4 people

Ingredients:

- 1/3 cup fresh orange juice
- 2 tablespoons balsamic vinegar
- 1 tablespoon extra-virgin olive oil
- salt and pepper to taste

Directions:

1. Place all ingredients in a bowl.
2. Whisk until well-combined.
3. Place in a small jar and shake well before using.
4. Keep inside the fridge for two days.

Nutrition: Calories: 43, Total Fat: 4g, Saturated Fat: 0.5g, Total Carbs: 4g, Net Carbs: 4g, Protein: 0.1g, Sugar: 1g, Fiber: 0g, Sodium: 73 mg, Potassium: 103mg

ANTI-INFLAMMATORY APPLESAUCE

PREPARATION: 10 min.
COOKING TIME: 15 min.
SERVING: 5 people

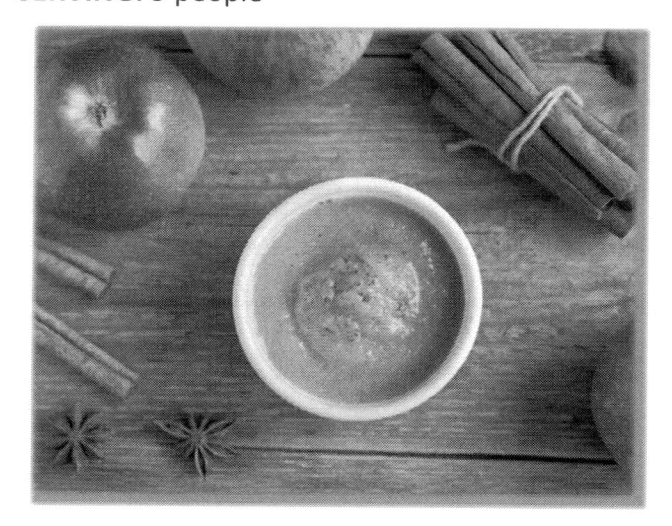

Ingredients:

- 12 organic apples, peeled, cored, and sliced
- 2 teaspoons cinnamon
- Water for steamer pot

Directions:

1. Pour water in a deep pan and place a steamer basket on top.
2. Place apples in the steamer and steam for 15 minutes until soft.
3. Place the apples in a food processor and add in cinnamon.
4. Pulse until smooth.
5. Place in containers and store in the fridge until ready to consume.

Nutrition: Calories: 287, Total Fat: 0.9g, Saturated Fat: 0.1g, Total Carbs: 76g, Net Carbs: 62g, Protein: 2g, Sugar: 56 g, Fiber: 14g, Sodium: 6mg, Potassium: 590mg

DRIED HERB RUB

PREPARATION: 5 min.
COOKING TIME: -
SERVING: 1 person

Ingredients:

- Dried thyme – 1 tbsp
- Dried oregano – 1 tbsp
- Dried parsley – 1 tbsp
- Dried basil – 2 tsp
- Ground coriander – 2 tsp
- Onion powder – 2 tsp
- Ground cumin – 1 tsp
- Garlic powder – 1 tsp
- Paprika – 1 tsp
- Cayenne pepper – ½ tsp

Directions:

1. Put all the ingredients into a blender and blend until smooth and mixed.
2. Store and use as needed.

Nutrition: Calories: 3, Fat: 0g, Carb: 1g, Phosphorus: 3mg, Potassium: 16mg, Sodium: 1mg, Protein: 0g

MEDITERRANEAN SEASONING

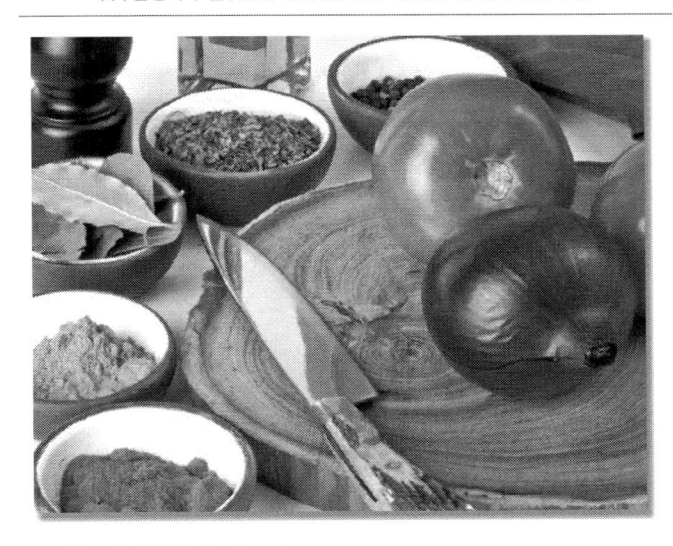

PREPARATION: 5 min.
COOKING TIME: -
SERVING: 1 person

Ingredients:

- Dried oregano – 2 tbsp
- Dried thyme – 1 tbsp
- Dried rosemary – 2 tsp, chopped
- Dried basil – 2 tsp
- Dried marjoram – 1 tsp
- Dried parsley flakes – 1 tsp

Directions:

1. In a bowl, mix all the ingredients.
2. Store in a container and use.

Nutrition: Calories: 1, Fat: 0g, Carb: 0g, Phosphorus: 1mg, Potassium: 6mg, Sodium: 0mg, Protein: 0g

HOT CURRY POWDER

PREPARATION: 5 min.
COOKING TIME: -
SERVING: 1 person

Ingredients:

- Ground cumin – ¼ cup
- Ground coriander – ¼ cup
- Turmeric – 3 tbsp
- Sweet paprika – 2 tbsp
- Ground Mustard – 2 tbsp
- Fennel powder – 1 tbsp
- Green chili powder - ½ tsp
- Ground cardamom – 2 tsp
- Ground cinnamon – 1 tsp
- Ground cloves – ½ tsp

Directions:

1. Put all in a blender and pulse until the ingredients are ground and well combined.

2. Store and use.

Nutrition: Calories: 19, Fat: 1g, Carb: 3g, Phosphorus: 24mg, Potassium: 93mg, Sodium: 5mg, Protein: 1g

CAJUN SEASONING

PREPARATION: 5 min.
COOKING TIME: -
SERVING: 1 person

Ingredients

- Sweet paprika – ½ cup
- Garlic powder – ¼ cup
- Onion powder – 3 tbsp
- Ground black pepper – 3 tbsp
- Dried oregano – 2 tbsp
- Cayenne pepper – 1 tbsp
- Dried thyme – 1 tbsp

Directions:

1. Put everything in a blender and pulse until the ingredients are ground and well combined.

2. Store and use.

Nutrition: Calories: 7 Fat: 0g Carb: 2g, Phosphorus: 8mg, Potassium: 40mg, Sodium: 1mg, Protein: 0g

RAS EL HANOUT

PREPARATION: 5 min.
COOKING TIME: -
SERVING: 1 person

Ingredients:

- Ground nutmeg – 2 tsp
- Ground coriander – 2 tsp
- Ground cumin – 2 tsp
- Turmeric – 2 tsp
- Cinnamon – 2 tsp
- Cardamom – 1 tsp
- Sweet paprika – 1 tsp
- Ground mace – 1 tsp
- Ground black pepper – 1 tsp
- Cayenne pepper – 1 tsp
- Ground allspice – ½ tsp
- Ground loves – ½ tsp

Directions:

1. In a bowl, mix everything until combined well.
2. Store and use.

Nutrition: Calories: 5, Fat: 0g, Carb: 1g, Phosphorus: 3mg, Potassium: 17mg, Sodium: 1mg, Protein: 0g

POULTRY SEASONING

PREPARATION: 5 min.
COOKING TIME: -
SERVING: 1 person

Ingredients:

- Ground thyme – 2 tbsp
- Ground marjoram – 2 tbsp
- Ground sage – 1 tbsp
- Ground celery seed – 1 tbs
- Ground rosemary - 1 tsp
- Ground black pepper -1 tsp

Directions:

1. In a bowl, mix everything until combined well.
2. Store and use.

Nutrition: Calories: 3 Fat: 0g, Carb: 0g, Phosphorus: 3mg, Potassium: 10mg, Sodium: 1mg, Protein: 0g

ADOBO SEASONING MIX

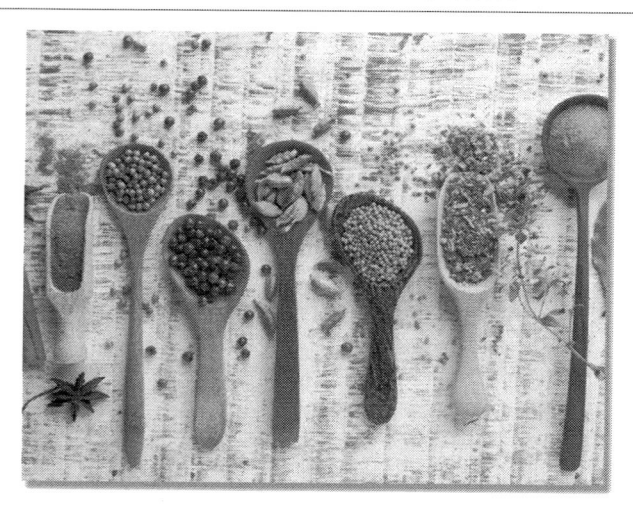

PREPARATION: 5 min.
COOKING TIME: -
SERVING: 1 person

Ingredients:

- Garlic powder – 4 tbsp
- Onion powder – 4 tbsp
- Ground cumin – 4 tbsp
- Dried oregano – 3 tbsp
- Ground black pepper – 3 tbsp
- Sweet paprika – 2 tbsp
- Ground chili powder – 2 tbsp
- Ground turmeric – 1 tbsp
- Ground coriander – 1 tbsp

Directions:

1. In a bowl, mix everything until well combined.
2. Store and use.

Nutrition: Calories: 8, Fat: 0g, Carb: 2g, Phosphorus: 9mg, Potassium: 38mg, Sodium: 12mg, Protein: 0g

HERBS DE PROVENCE

PREPARATION: 5 min.
COOKING TIME: -
SERVING: 1 person

Ingredients:

- Dried thyme – ½ cup
- Dried marjoram – 3 tbsp
- Dried savory – 3 tbsp
- Dried rosemary – 2 tbsp
- Dried lavender flowers - 2 tsp
- Ground fennel – 1 tsp

Directions:

1. Put everything in a blender and mix well.
2. Store and use.

Nutrition: Calories: 3, Fat: 0g, Carb: 1g, Phosphorus: 2mg, Potassium: 9mg, Sodium: 0mg, Protein: 0g

HONEY MUSTARD

PREPARATION: 5 min.
COOKING TIME: -
SERVING: 1 person

Ingredients:

- ½ teaspoon onion powder
- 1 teaspoon garlic powder
- ¼ teaspoon ground white pepper
- 1 tablespoon ground mustard
- ¼ cup honey
- ¼ cup white vinegar
- ¾ cup olive oil

Directions:

1. Add all the ingredients in the order in a food processor or blender, except for oil and honey, and pulse at medium speed until blended.

2. Slowly blend in oil until incorporated and then mix in honey, 1 tablespoon at a time, until mustard reaches to desired sweetness.

3. Transfer the mustard into a bowl, then cover the bowl and store for up to 2 months in the refrigerator.

4. Serve when desired.

Nutrition: 108 Cal; 4.9 g Carb; 0 g Protein; 10.2 g Fat, 0.3 g Fiber; 0.5 mg Sodium; 11.7 mg Potassium; 25 mg Phosphorus

PICKLES

PREPARATION: 10 min.
COOKING TIME: -
SERVING: 58 people

Ingredients:

- 5 English cucumbers, sliced
- 1 teaspoon ground black pepper
- 2 cups brown sugar
- 1/2 teaspoon dry mustard
- 1 teaspoon ground turmeric
- 1 1/2 cups red wine vinegar
- 2 teaspoons celery seed
- 2 tablespoons dill weed
- 1 1/2 cups apple cider vinegar
- 1 bunch fresh dill
- 2 cups white wine vinegar

Directions:

1. Prepare the cucumbers - slice them, then layer them evenly in pint jars and evenly fill the jars with black pepper, mustard, turmeric, celery, dill weed, and dill.

2. Pour all the kinds of vinegar in a pitcher, add brown sugar, and stir well until sugar has dissolved.

3. Pour the vinegar mixture into pint jars, leaving some space at the top, and then cover the jars with lids.

4. Place the jars in the refrigerator and store them for up to six months.

Nutrition: 30 Cal; 7 g Carb; 0 g Protein; 0 g Fat, 2.5 g Fiber; 1 mg Sodium; 15 mg Potassium; 2 mg Phosphorus

TERIYAKI SAUCE

PREPARATION: 5 min.
COOKING TIME: -
SERVING: 1 person

Ingredients:

- 1 ½ teaspoon minced garlic
- 1/2 cup brown sugar
- 1/4 teaspoon ground ginger
- 2 tablespoons Chinese sweet rice wine
- 2 tablespoons sesame oil
- 1 cup soy sauce, sodium-reduced

Directions:

1. Take a small saucepan, place it over low heat, add all the ingredients in it, stir until just mixed, and cook for 5 to 10 minutes until the sugar has dissolved.
2. Then let the sauce cool completely, pour it into an air-tight glass container, cover with the lid, then keep it in the refrigerator and store for up to 1 month.
3. Serve when desired.

Nutrition: 29 Cal; 5 g Carb; 1 g Protein; 0 g Fat, 1 g Fiber; 308 mg Sodium; 1 mg Potassium; 308 mg Phosphorus

ALFREDO SAUCE

PREPARATION: 5 min.
COOKING TIME: 15 min.
SERVING: 1 ¾ cup

Ingredients:

- 3 tablespoons all-purpose flour
- ½ teaspoon minced garlic
- 1/4 teaspoon ground nutmeg
- 1/4 cup olive oil
- 1 tablespoon lemon juice
- 2 cups of rice milk, unsweetened
- 4 ounces cream cheese, sodium-reduced
- 1/3 cup grated parmesan cheese, sodium-reduced

Directions:

1. Take a large skillet, place it over medium heat, add oil in it and when hot, add flour and whisk until well mixed.
2. Then stir in garlic and pour in milk, whisking continuously until smooth and bring the mixture to boil.
3. Continue cooking the sauce for 5 to 10 minutes until it has thickened to desired consistency or reduced by half, then stir in cream cheese until combined and remove the pan from heat.
4. Add remaining ingredients into the sauce, stir well until mixed, and let cool for 10 minutes.
5. Ladle sauce over broiled rice, steamed vegetables cooked chicken, etc. and serve.

Nutrition: 173 Cal; 9 g Carb; 3 g Protein; 14 g Fat, 2 g Fiber; 142 mg Sodium; 32 mg Potassium; 75 mg Phosphorus

TOMATO SALSA

PREPARATION: 5 min.
COOKING TIME: -
SERVING: 1 person

Ingredients:

- 2 green onions, chopped
- 1 medium green bell pepper, cored, chopped
- 1 jalapeño pepper, chopped
- 4 Roma tomatoes, chopped
- 1/2 bunch fresh cilantro, chopped
- 1 ½ teaspoon minced garlic
- 1 tablespoon dried oregano
- 1/2 teaspoon cumin

Directions:

1. Add all the ingredients in the order in a blender or food processor and pulse for 2 minutes until mixed well and chunky.
2. Tip the salsa in an 8-ounce pint jar, cover it and let cool for 3 hours.
3. Store the salsa for up to two weeks in a refrigerator and serve with tortilla chips.

Nutrition: 14 Cal; 2 g Carb; 1 g Protein; 1 g Fat, 0 g Fiber; 4 mg Sodium; 117 mg Potassium; 14 mg Phosphorus

FAJITA FLAVOR MARINADE

PREPARATION: 5 min.
COOKING TIME: -
SERVING: 1 person

Ingredients

- 1 jalapeño pepper, finely diced
- 1 medium grapefruit, juiced
- 1/4 teaspoon garlic powder
- 2 medium limes, juiced
- 3 tablespoons olive oil
- 1 medium orange, juiced

Directions:

1. Take a medium bowl, place all the ingredients in it, and stir well until combined.
2. Pour the marinade over chicken or vegetables, toss until well coated, and let marinate for 1 hour.
3. Drizzle the marinade over chicken or vegetables and cook as instructed in the recipe.

Nutrition: 33 Cal; 2 g Carb; 0 g Protein; 2.8 g Fat, 1 g Fiber; 0 mg Sodium; 42 mg Potassium; 5 mg Phosphorus.

GARLIC-HERB SEASONING

PREPARATION: 5 min.
COOKING TIME: -
SERVING: 1 person

Ingredients:

- 2 teaspoons garlic powder
- 1 teaspoon powdered lemon rind
- 1 teaspoon dried oregano
- 1 teaspoon dried basil

Directions:

1. Add all the ingredients in the order in a food processor or blender and blend at medium speed until combined.
2. Tip the mixture in an air-tight glass container, add a few grains of rice to keep the mixture from clumping and store until ready to use.

Nutrition: Cal 12, Carb 3g; Protein 0g; Fat 0g, Fiber 1g; Sodium 1 mg; Potassium 47mg; Phosphorus 16mg.

LIME CARIBBEAN DRESSING

PREPARATION: 5 min.
COOKING TIME: -
SERVING: 1 person

Ingredients:

- 2 teaspoons pineapple preserves
- 3 drops hot sauce
- 2 fresh limes
- 1/3 cup low-fat mayonnaise

Directions:

1. Zest one of the limes and set aside
2. Juice both limes into a small bowl
3. Add mayonnaise and pineapple preserves to lime juice and whisk together until well blended
4. Fold in lime zest. Stir in a few drops of hot sauce if desired

Nutrition: Cal 75; Carb 7g; Protein 0g; Fat 5g, Fiber 0,2g; Sodium 127g; Potassium 31mg; Phosphorus 12mg; Cholesterol 5mg; Calcium 3mg.

BONUS CHAPTER:
WORKOUT FOR KIDNEY PATIENTS:
KEEPING ACTIVE DESPITE KIDNEY DISEASE

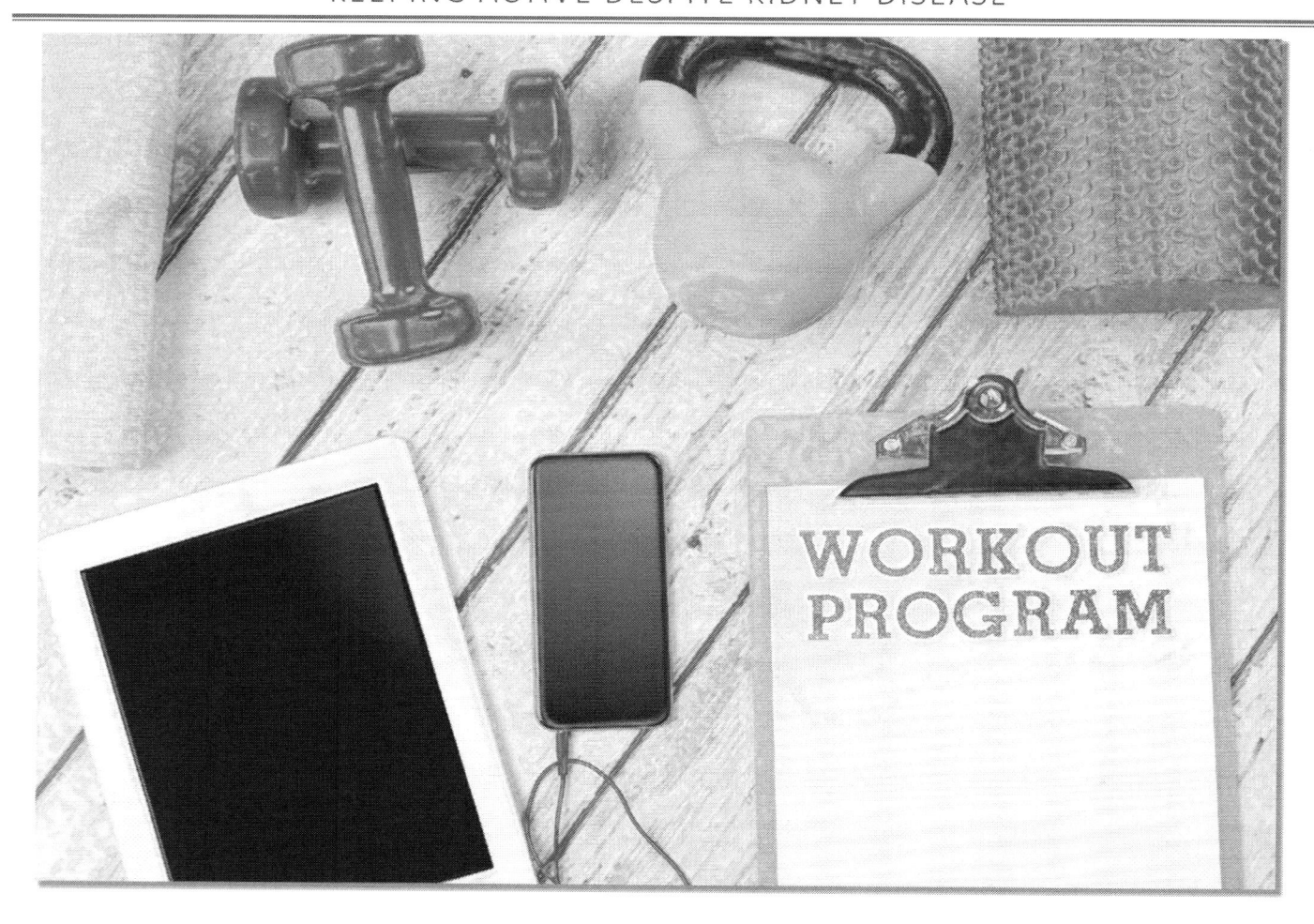

Kidney Disease is a condition that affects the kidneys. It can be caused by several factors, such as diabetes, high blood pressure, and other chronic conditions.

It can be difficult to stay fit if you have kidney disease because your kidneys are not functioning properly. This means that your body is not able to remove waste products from your blood efficiently. Therefore you need to limit the amount of exercise you do and make sure it's low-impact.

In many cases, kidney disease can be managed with lifestyle changes such as diet and exercise. Exercise is important for people with kidney disease because it helps maintain muscle mass and bone strength, which are often lost when someone has a chronic illness.

There are many benefits to exercise, and it can be a great way to help manage your CKD. Exercise for CKD is not about taking on high-impact or high-intensity workouts. It's about finding ways to be active throughout the day.

Exercise can help improve your overall health and well-being, which may lead to better management of your CKD.

Regular physical activity has been shown to improve kidney function in people with chronic kidney disease, reduce their risk of developing complications and reduce their need for medications.

One of the most common symptoms is fatigue, which is caused by the buildup of toxins in the body. Exercise has been shown to help reduce this symptom and improve overall health.

There are many exercise options for people with kidney disease, but some are better than others.

Swimming, for example, is a great option because it doesn't put any pressure on your joints or muscles, and it doesn't require you to be on your feet for long periods.

Yoga is also a good choice because it's easy on your joints and muscles - and many poses can be modified to accommodate those with physical limitations.

Start slowly, with gentle exercises like **walking** or **stretching** that don't strain the kidneys - Take time to warm up before exercising and cool down afterward - Drink plenty of fluids before, during, and after exercising - Wear comfortable shoes that provide good arch support.

You can do all of the following **four types of exercises** inside the comfort of your own home. Let's go over each one individually*.

EXERCISES TO INCREASE FLEXIBILITY*

These exercises test your joints' capacity to continue moving in the manner required for physical activity. Basic stretches, yoga, and Tai Chi are a few examples of flexibility activities that might significantly reduce your risk of injury when performing exercises.

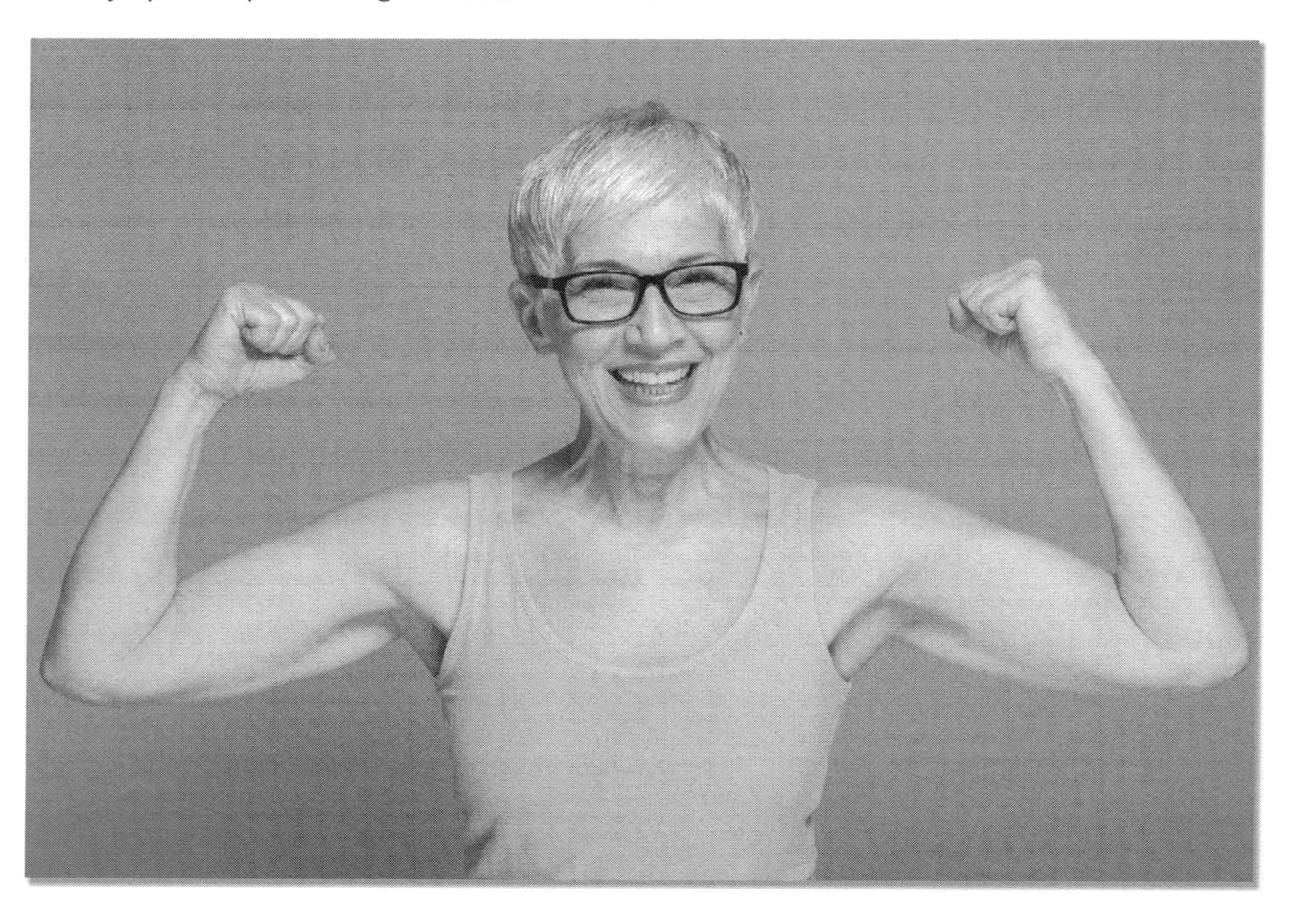

Some examples of flexibility exercises that may be beneficial for people with CKD include:

- **Gentle stretching:** This can help improve range of motion and reduce muscle stiffness. Start by standing up straight and slowly reaching for the sky with both hands. Hold for a few seconds and then release. Repeat this several times.

- **Yoga:** Yoga is a form of exercise that involves a series of poses and stretches that can help improve flexibility and relaxation. There are many different types of yoga, so it's important to find one that is suitable for your fitness level and abilities.

- **Tai chi:** This is a gentle, low-impact exercise that involves slow, flowing movements that can help improve flexibility and balance. Tai chi is often recommended for people with CKD because it can be done at a slow pace and is gentle on the joints.

SHOULDER ROTATION

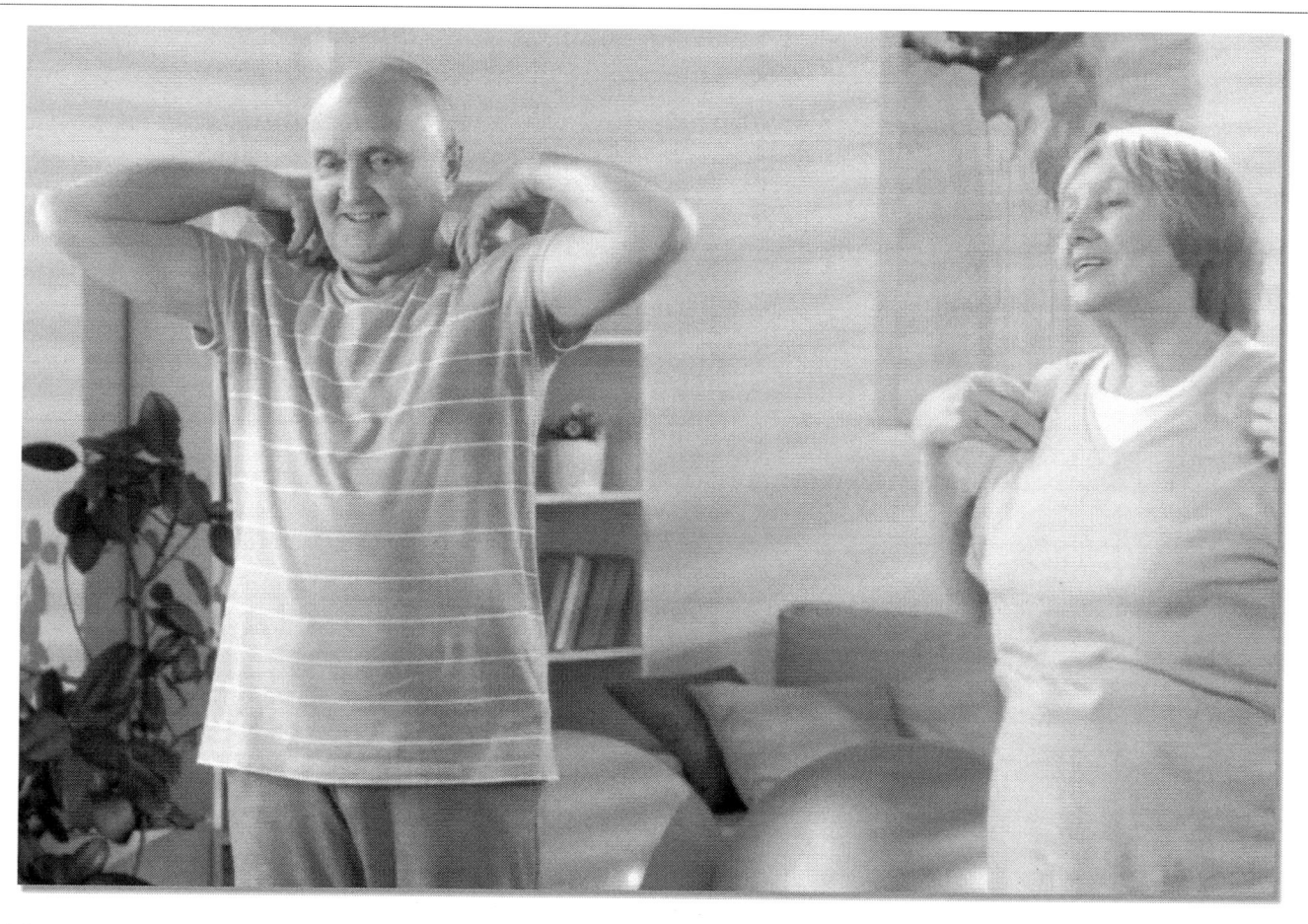

Shoulder rotation exercises can be beneficial because they can help improve flexibility and range of motion in the shoulders. This can help reduce stiffness and pain, and improve overall mobility and function.

One simple shoulder rotation exercise that is suitable for CKD is to stand up straight and hold your arms out to the sides at shoulder height.

Step 1: Slowly rotate your shoulders forward in a circular motion, making sure to keep your arms straight.

Step 2: Do 10-15 rotations in one direction, and then repeat in the opposite direction.

CHEST AND UPPER BACK STRETCH

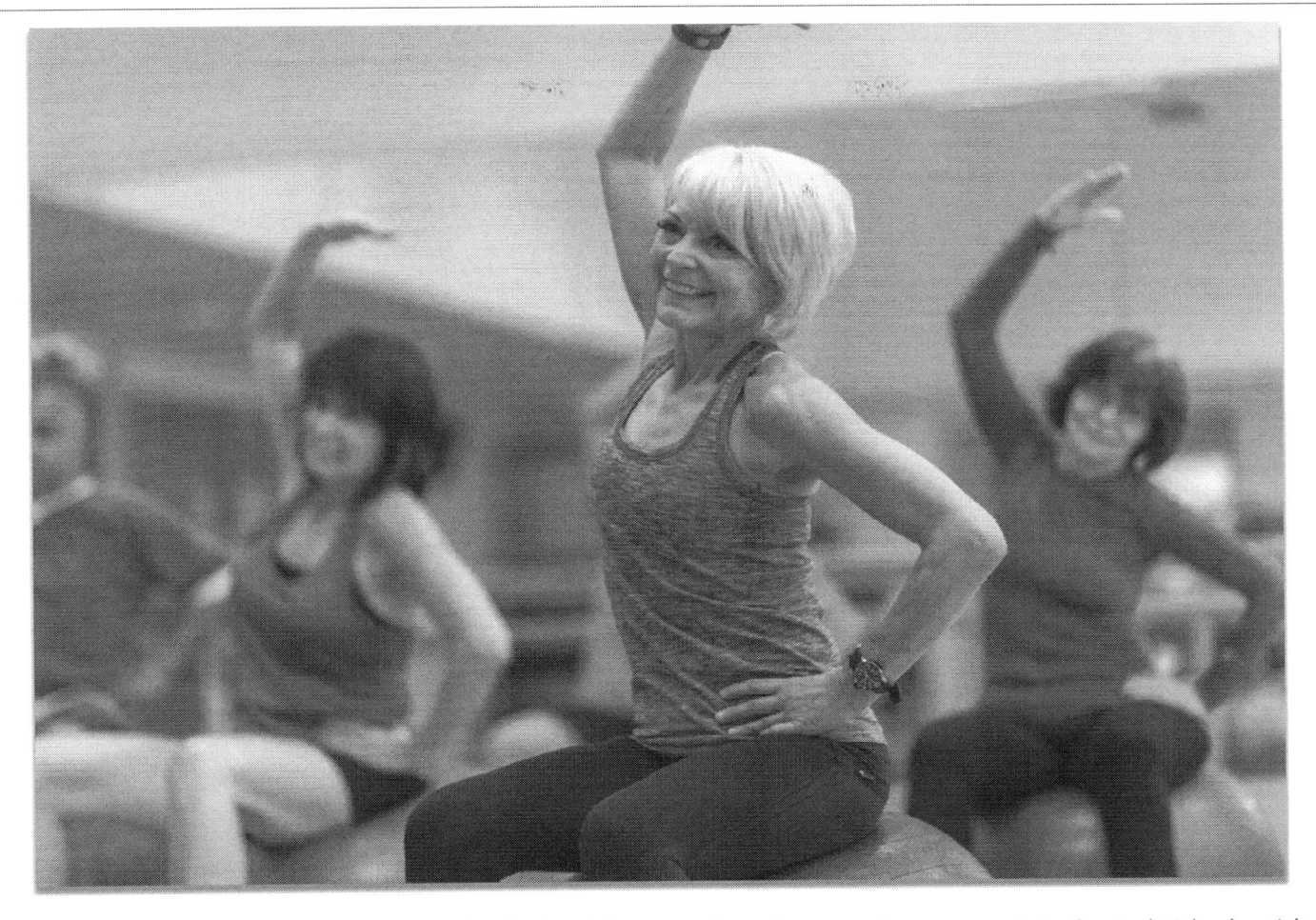

There are several chest and upper back shoulder exercises that may be appropriate for individuals with CKD. It is important to start with **low-intensity exercises** and gradually increase the intensity as tolerated.

Here are just a few examples:

1. Stand with your feet shoulder-width apart, hands behind your back, and palms facing out.
2. Lift your arms up and back, keeping your elbows straight.
3. Hold this position for 15-30 seconds, then release.

You can also do this stretch while seated:

1. Sit with your feet flat on the ground and your arms behind your back, palms facing out.
2. Lift your arms up and back, keeping your elbows straight.
3. Hold this position for 15-30 seconds, then release.

It is important to keep your core engaged and your shoulders relaxed while doing this stretch. You should feel a stretch in your chest and upper back. If the stretch is too intense, you can bring your arms back slightly to reduce the intensity. Remember to breathe deeply and slowly while holding the stretch.

LEG STRETCHES

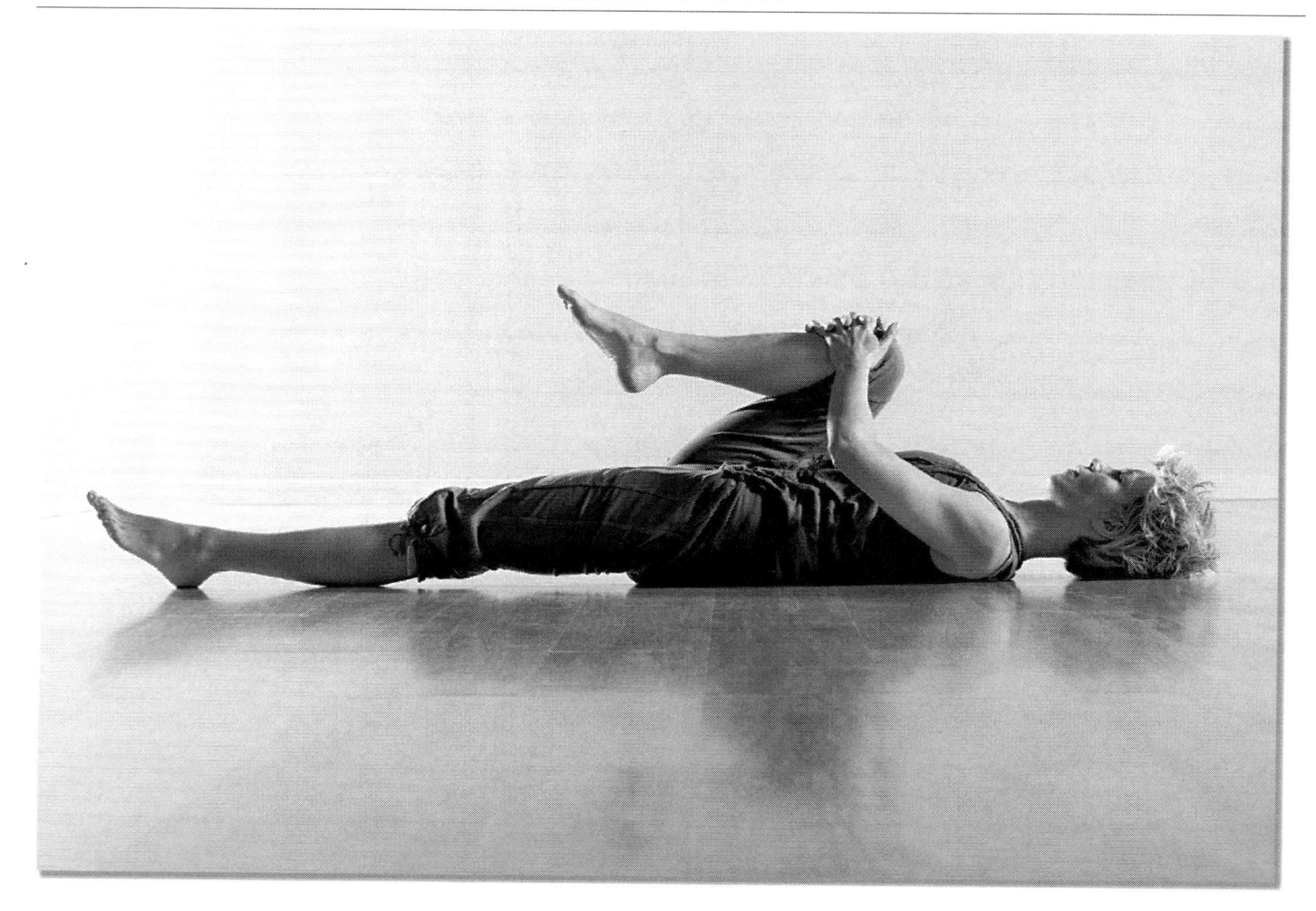

Step 1: Laying on your back, fold your right leg while keeping your left leg straight.

Step 2: Put both of your hands below your right leg, then draw your thigh toward your chest, and keep this position for 15 to 30 seconds.

Step 3: Repeat with your left leg.

AEROBIC EXERCISES*

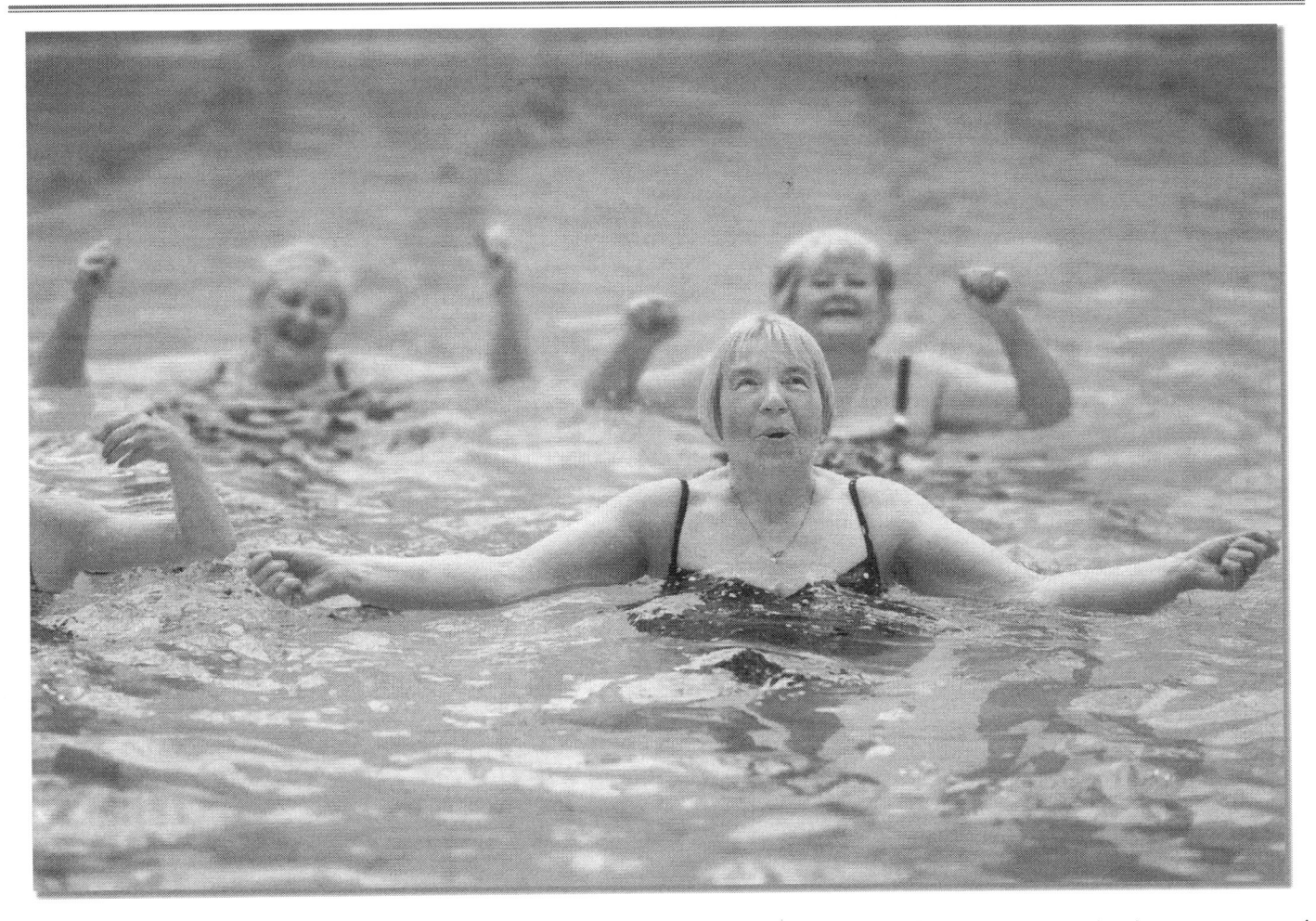

Aerobic exercise, also known as cardiovascular exercise, is any activity that increases the heart rate and breathing rate for an extended period of time. Examples of aerobic exercise include walking, jogging, cycling, and swimming. These types of exercises can be especially beneficial for individuals with CKD, as they can help to improve heart and lung function, reduce the risk of heart disease, and improve overall physical function.

People with CKD should do 150 minutes of moderate or 75 minutes of intense exercise per week. They should also talk to their doctor before starting an exercise plan, as they may need special precautions or changes based on how severe their CKD is and other things.

It is also important for individuals with CKD to stay hydrated during and after exercise, as the kidneys may not be able to efficiently remove excess fluids from the body. This can be especially important for individuals on dialysis, as dehydration can lead to complications during treatment. It is generally recommended to drink at least 8-12 cups of fluids per day, and to drink more during and after exercise to replace any fluids lost through sweat.

Here is a typical walking schedule you may follow:

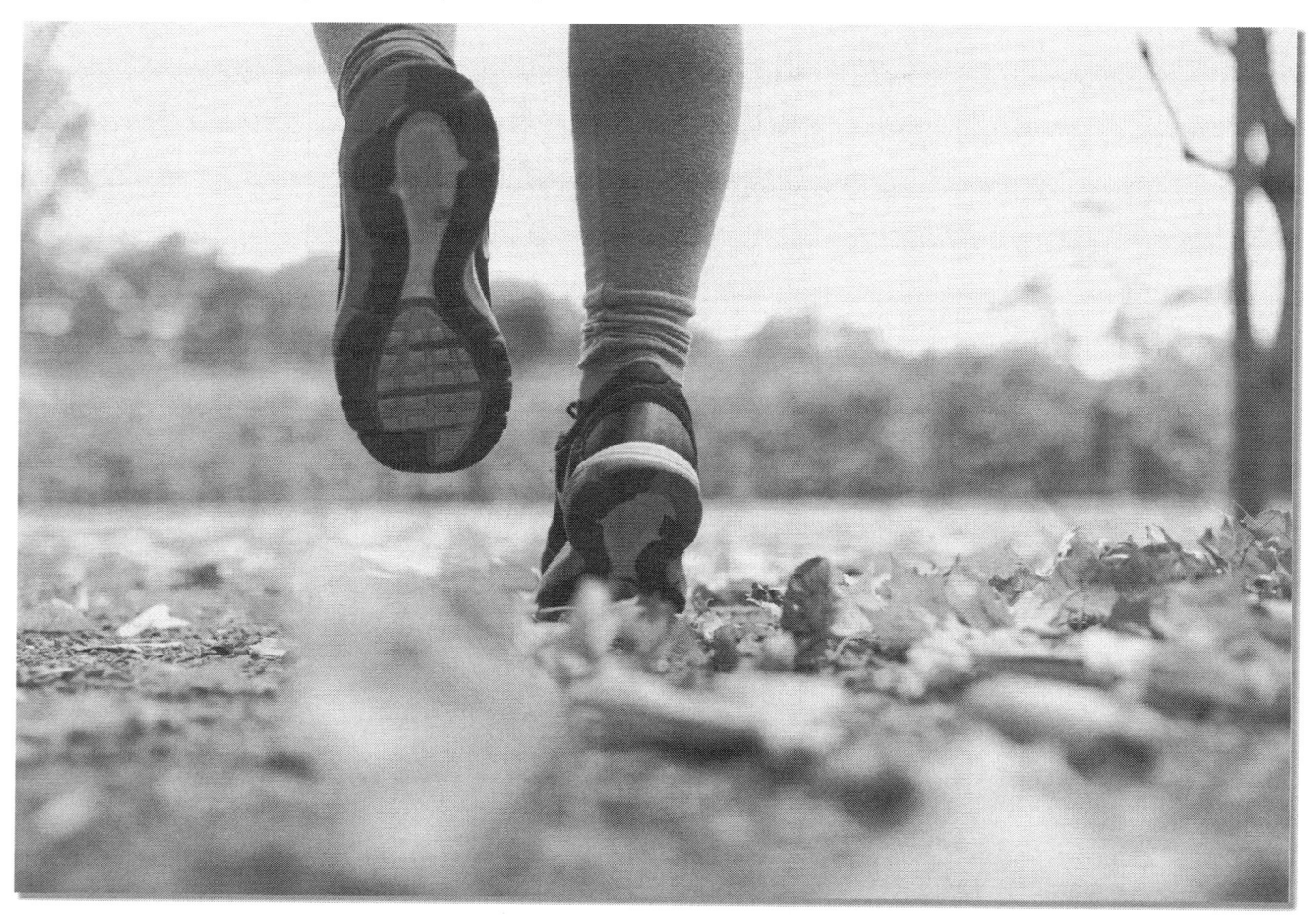

Step 1: Start by walking steadily but slowly for **10 minutes, five days a week**

Step 2: As you feel confident, **increase** your **daily** walking time **to 10 minutes** and then, every other day, **to 20 minutes** at a faster rate.

Step 3: Try to **extend** your time to **30 minutes** every other day for a month.

STRENGTH EXERCISES*

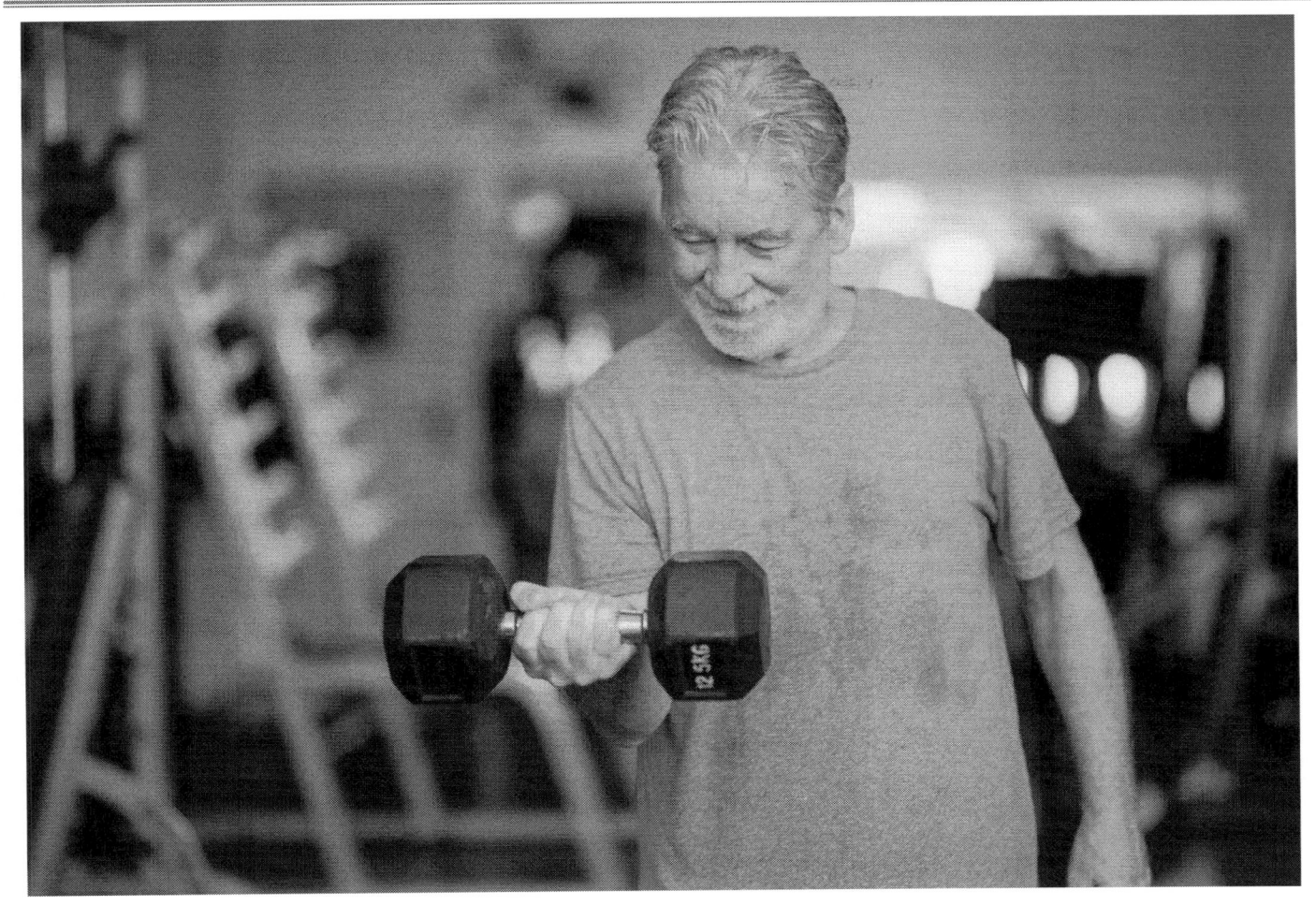

Strengthening exercises, on the other hand, require the use of muscles to perform activities. A few examples are Pilates, kettlebells, medicine balls, resistance bands, and weightlifting with dumbbells.

Here is a couple of basic home exercises routine for developing muscle strength:

BICEP CURL:

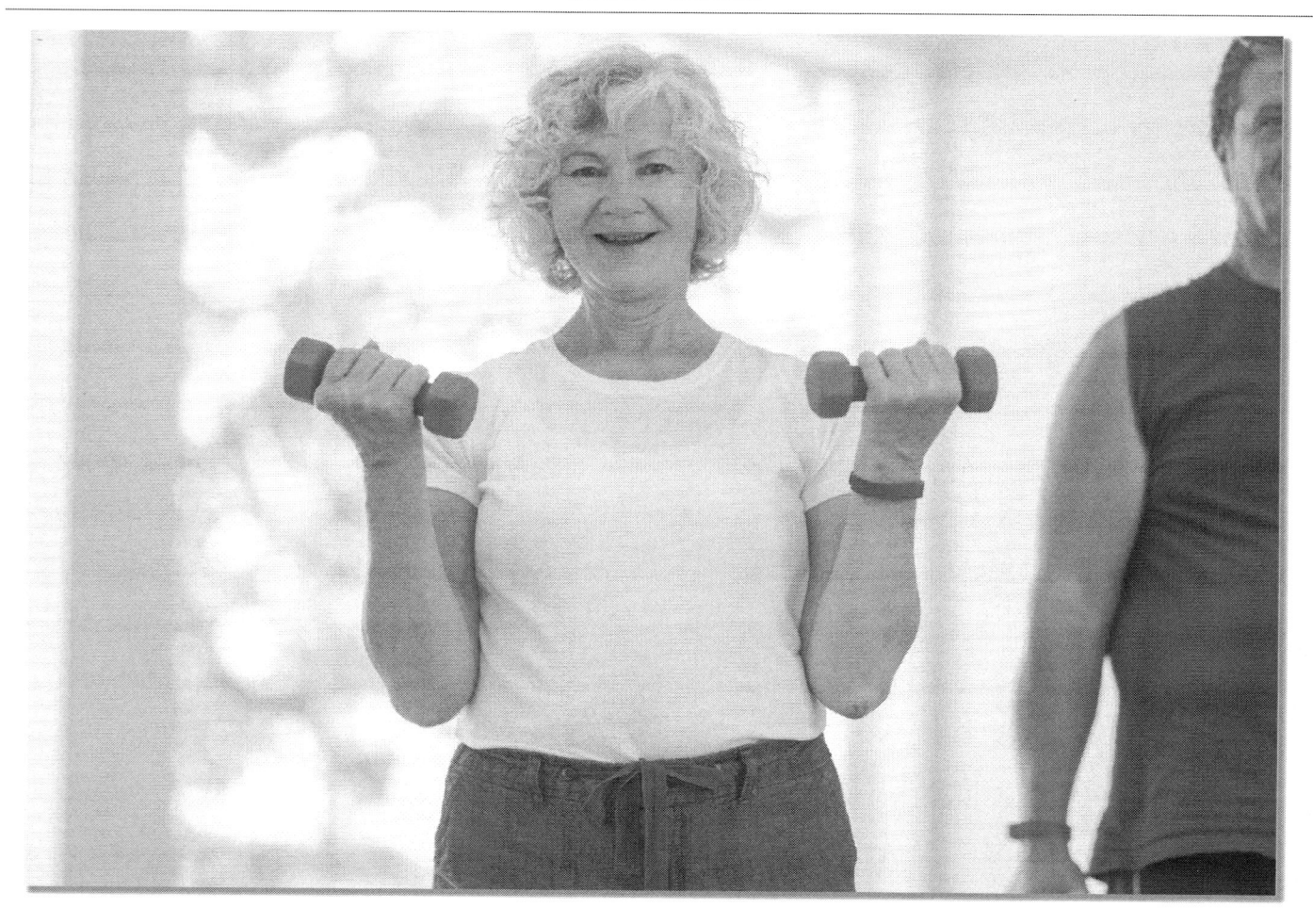

To perform bicep curls do the following steps:

Step 1: stand with your feet shoulder-width apart and hold a pair of dumbbells at your sides with your palms facing forward.

Step 2: Keeping your elbows close to your body, slowly curl the dumbbells up towards your shoulders, then lower them back down to the starting position.

You can do this exercise seated or standing, and you can use a variety of grip widths and hand positions to target different muscle fibers in your biceps.

It's important to start with a light weight and gradually increase the resistance as you get stronger. It's crucial to perform the exercises correctly to prevent injuries and make the most out of your workout.

LEG LIFT

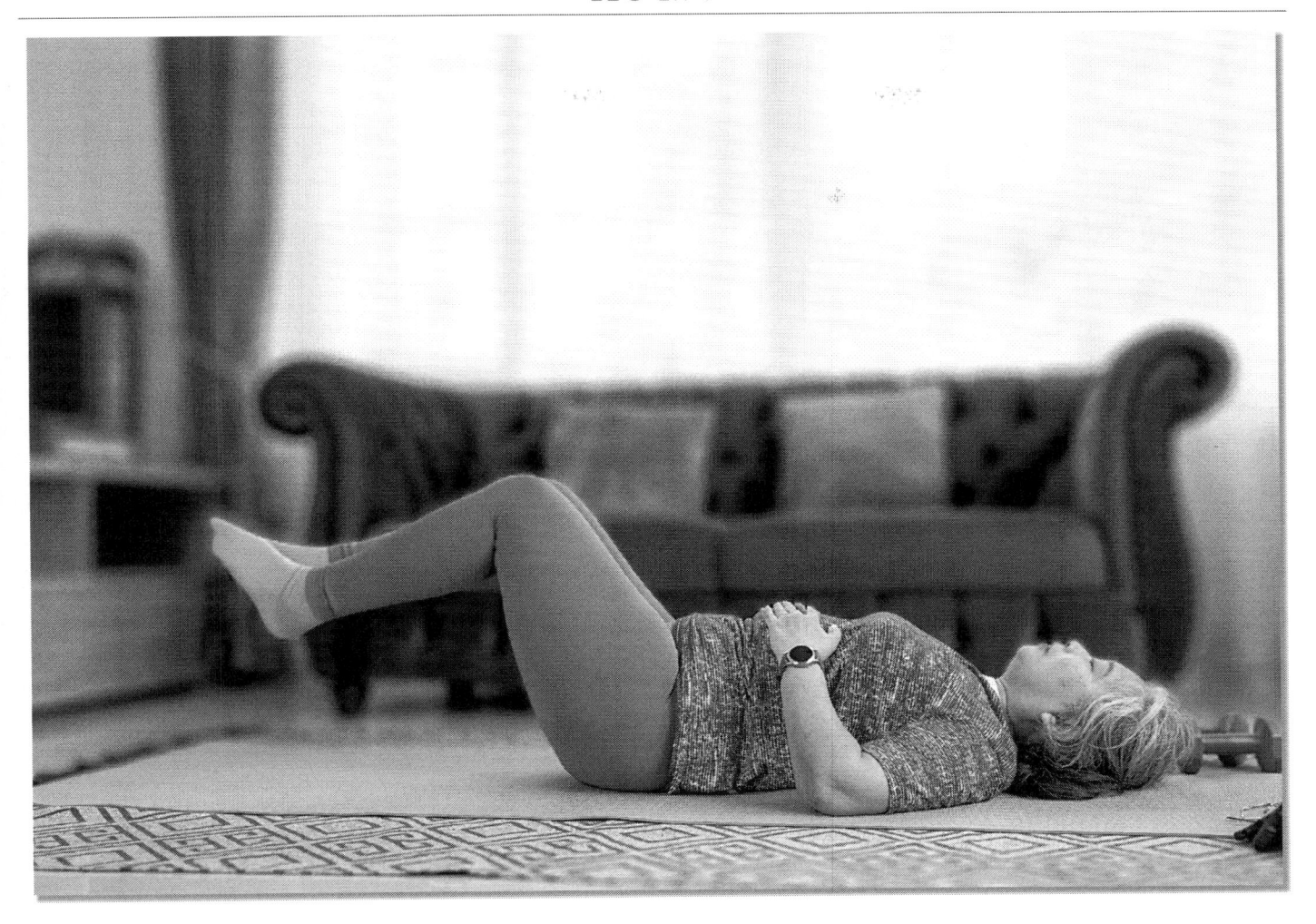

There are several variations of leg lifts that can be performed, including **standing** leg lifts, **seated** leg lifts, and leg lifts while **lying on your back** or **stomach**.

To perform leg lifts:

Step 1: Lie on your back on a flat surface with your arms by your sides and your legs straight.

Step 2: Slowly raise one leg straight up and then bring it back down. You can do this for both legs at the same time or alternate them.

You can also make the exercise more or less challenging by lifting your leg higher or lower from the ground.

It's important to start with a small range of motion and gradually increase the difficulty as you get stronger.

TIPS AND PRECAUTIONS TO BE CONSIDERED WHEN EXERCISING FOR KIDNEY HEALTH PROBLEMS

What are the signs that I should stop exercising?

If you experience any of the following during an exercise session, **stop immediately**:

You feel chest pains, irregular or rapid heartbeats, nausea, leg cramps, light-headedness, or dizziness, as well as other symptoms.

What about Fluid Intake?

Exercise can cause heavy sweating, so patients with CKD may think they need to drink more water.

In situations like this, lost fluids may need to be replaced. But in any case, we advise you to consult with your physician.

---

*It is important to consult with a healthcare provider before starting any new exercise program, especially if you have CKD. A healthcare provider can recommend specific exercises and provide guidance on how to properly perform them to avoid injury.

In general, people with CKD may need to modify their exercise program to accommodate their physical limitations and any fluid or electrolyte imbalances they may be experiencing. It's important to pay attention to your body's signals during exercise and stop if you experience any unusual symptoms such as chest pain, shortness of breath, dizziness, or muscle cramps.

CONCLUSION

Kidney disease is a serious condition that needs to be dealt with promptly. Therefore, It is recommended that you use this book in conjunction with healthcare professionals to help control the symptoms and complications of renal disease.

To avoid these complications, this book is a great starting guide to maintain a good health.

This book is my hard work to help patients to maintain good health, along with diet plans. There are many schemes to provide a good number of proteins. These schemes include egg white, egg yolk, egg white+egg yolk combined, cheese, curd and so on.

This guide provides a range of delicious, healthy, and easy-to-prepare meals. You'll find that there's no need for special ingredients or hard-to-find spices when cooking kidney-friendly dishes with taste that's out of this world!

This cookbook contains a selection of both sweet and savory recipes with an emphasis on lean proteins, complex carbohydrates, and vitamin-rich vegetables. Whether you're managing renal disease or simply looking for healthier meal options, this cookbook contains easy-to-cook recipes that are all low in potassium, phosphorus and protein.

I hope the information I have provided in this book has been helpful to you or your family.

Finally, if you think this information is helpful, please leave your honest review on Amazon. This way many more people will be able to benefit from it.

Thank you very much.

CONVERSION TABLES

Volume Equivalents (Liquid)

US STANDARD	US STANDARD (OUNCES)	METRIC (APPROXIMATE)
2 tablespoons	1 fl. ounce.	30 mL
1/4 cup	2 fl. ounce.	60 mL
1/2 cup	4 fl. ounce.	120 mL
1 cup	8 fl. ounce.	240 mL
11/2 cups	12 fl. ounce.	355 mL
2 cups or 1 pint	16 fl. ounce.	475 mL
4 cups or 1 quart	32 fl. ounce.	1 L
1 gallon	128 fl. ounce.	4 L

Volume Equivalents (Dry)

US STANDARD	METRIC (APPROXIMATE)
1/4 teaspoon	1 mL
1/2 teaspoon	2 mL
1 teaspoon	5 mL
1 tablespoon	15 mL
1/4 cup	59 mL
cup	79 mL
1/2 cup	118 mL
1 cup	177 mL

Oven Temperatures

FAHRENHEIT (F)	CELSIUS (C) (APPROXIMATE)
250°F	120 °C
300°F	150°C
325°F	165°C
350°F	180°C
375°F	190°C
400°F	200°C
425°F	220°C
450°F	230°C

Weight Equivalents

US STANDARD	METRIC (APPROXIMATE)
1/2 ounce	15 g
1 ounce	30 g
2 ounces	60 g
4 ounces	115 g
8 ounces	225 g
12 ounces	340 g
16 ounces or 1 pound	455 g

SHOPPING RESOURCES

It is best to consult with your doctor or dietician to come up with a proper shopping list when trying to live with chronic kidney disease. Below is a compiled list of items that can be bought at the grocery store and are considered kidney-friendly options. Most of the items on the list can be bought at any local grocery store, but remember that fresh is always the best option. Try visiting your local farmers market for fresher alternatives.

Make sure that you are asking about growing situations when purchasing that way because some fertilizers can introduce extra phosphates into the food. You want to keep the fruits or vegetables that you are buying as close to the principle of "farm to table" as you can. Fresher is better, but if you are stuck with cans, make sure there is nothing added to them, and they are as close to raw form as possible.

Even though these are just suggestions, it is always important for you to look at your labels and become acquainted with what the words mean and the servings you are looking at. Something may be low in sodium, but the serving size may be so small it doesn't make it worth it.

Sometimes practicing self-control when using any kind of lifestyle change can be hard at first, so when starting out, it is important to carefully lay out all of the things that you are buying and cooking so that you can hold yourself accountable. Use the compilation below to make food conscious and kidney conscious choices.

Juices
- Apricot
- Cranberry
- Cran-Apple
- Cran-Raspberry
- Grape
- Grapefruit
- Lemon
- Lemonade
- Papaya
- Pear
- Pineapple

Other
- Coffee
- Club Soda
- Clear and Caffeine Soda Drinks
- Cream Soda
- Ginger Ale
- Fresh Brewed Teas

Condiments/Sauces
- Chili Sauce
- BBQ
- Cornstarch
- Corn Syrup
- Mayonnaise or Salad Dressing
- Mustard
- Cream Cheese
- Honey
- Dry Tapioca
- Jam
- Jelly
- Ketchup
- Margarine
- Sugar Substitute
- Marmalade
- Taco Sauce
- Vinegar
- Worcestershire Sauce

- Steak Sauce

Sweet Treats

- Lemon Flavored Cakes and Cookies
- Angel Food Cake
- Chewing Gum
- Vanilla Wafers
- Hard Candies

Meat (Fresh)

- Beef
- Lamb
- Chicken
- Turkey
- Veal
- Pork
- Wild Caught Game (Like deer)

Seafood

- Fish (Fresh or Frozen)
- Salmon
- Shellfish
- Lobster
- Crab
- Tuna (canned in water)

Egg Substitutes

- **Tofu**

Dairy

- Milk (limited to .5 cup a day)
- Non-Dairy Creamers
- Non-Dairy Whipped Dessert Topping

Milk Alternatives

- Unenriched Almond
- Unenriched Rice
- Unenriched Soy

Grains/Bread/Cereals (No Whole Wheat Options)

- Bagels
- Dinner Rolls
- Flour Tortillas
- English Muffins
- Hamburger/Hot Dog Buns
- Rice Cakes
- Pita Bread
- Sourdough
- Rye
- Melba Toasts
- Cereals that do not include dried fruits, nuts, or granola
- Cream of Wheat
- Cream of Rice
- Grits

Crackers

- Animal Crackers
- Graham Crackers (Honey or Cinnamon)
- Oyster
- Rusk
- Low-Sodium Brown
- Low-Sodium or Unsalted Saltines
- Unsalted Pretzels
- Wheat Thins (Low-Sodium)

Pasta and Alternatives

- Couscous
- Lightly salted popcorn or unsalted popcorn
- Macaroni
- Spaghetti
- White Rice
- Egg Noodles

Fruit
- Cherries
- Apples
- Applesauce
- Clementine Oranges
- Apricots
- Lemons
- Blackberries
- Boysenberries
- Cranberries
- Grapes
- Grapefruit
- Limes
- Passion Fruit
- Peaches
- Pears
- Mandarin Oranges
- Pineapples
- Strawberries
- Raspberries
- Plums
- Tangerines

Vegetables
- Bean Sprouts
- Alfalfa Sprouts
- Bell Peppers (All Colors)
- Asparagus
- Cauliflower
- Bamboo Shoots
- Arugula
- Broccoli
- Cabbage
- Carrots
- Celery
- Chives
- Collard Greens
- Egg Plant
- Cucumber
- Lettuce
- Leeks
- Kale
- Mushrooms
- Okra
- Onion
- Peas
- Spinach
- Spaghetti Squash
- Zucchini
- Yellow Squash
- Radishes
- Turnips

Seasonings and Herbs
- Allspice
- Cloves
- Cinnamon
- Basil
- Bay Leaf
- Chili Powder
- Celery Seed
- Dry Mustard
- Cilantro
- Curry
- Cumin
- Marjoram
- Dill
- Extracts (Almond, Vanilla, Orange, Maple, Lemon, Peppermint)
- Fennel
- Sesame Seeds
- Garlic
- Ginger
- Paprika
- Mrs. Dash (Salt-Free and Low Sodium seasoning alternative)
- Nutmeg
- Pepper
- Oregano
- Parsley
- Rosemary
- Sage
- Thyme

THINGS TO AVOID ON A RENAL DIET

- Sodas that are dark in color
- Avocado
- Whole wheat bread and pasta
- Brown rice
- Bananas
- Processed meats (lunchmeats, hotdogs, and bacon)
- Pickles
- Olives
- Relish
- Prepackaged meals

It cannot be reiterated enough that you need to be reading all the labels of the foods you are buying. Doing your own research before grocery shopping is your first line of defense in living a true kidney-friendly life. This has laid out the information; all you have to do is put it to work for you. Make sure you are keeping an inventory of what you have and what you don't have because being proactive in your diet can help keep you from making an eating mistake in a pinch.

Most of these items should have a place in your pantry or refrigerator. It is important that you keep up on your renal diet, and there is nothing to lose by including your family in the diet. It is never too early to start living a lifestyle that can improve your quality of life.

REFERENCES

Renal Diet: How to Use Diet to Prevent Dialysis and Chronic Kidney Disease *(CKD). -* (*Renal Diet Cookbook Book 1*) by Emily Stevens

Renal Diet Cookbook for the Newly Diagnosed: The Complete Guide to Managing Kidney Disease and Avoiding Dialysis - by Susan Zogheib

The Complete Renal Diet Cookbook for Beginners: Low Sodium, Low Potassium & Low Phosphorus Renal Diet Recipes - by Viktoria McCartney

Renal Diet Cookbook for Beginners 2020: Only Low Sodium, Low Potassium, and Low Phosphorus Healthy Recipes to Control Your Kidney Disease (CKD) and Avoid Dialysis of Kidney - by Tina Cooper

Renal Diet Plan and Cookbook: The Optimal Nutrition Guide to Manage Kidney Disease - by Susan Zogheib RD LDN

Renal Diet Cookbook: The Low Sodium, Low Potassium, Healthy Kidney Cookbook - by Rockridge Press & Susan Zogheib

RECIPE INDEX

BREAKFAST 33

- Peach Berry Parfait 34
- Open-Faced Bagel Breakfast Sandwich 34
- Bulgur Bowl with Strawberries and Walnuts 35
- Overnight Oats Three Ways 35
- Buckwheat Pancakes 36
- Apple and Cinnamon French Toast Strata 37
- Broccoli Basil Quiche 37
- Asparagus Frittata 38
- Poached Eggs with Cilantro Butter 39
- Green Breakfast Soup 39
- Tasty Pancakes 40
- Slow Cooked Oats 40
- Papaya Orange Smoothie 41
- Brown Muffins 41
- Easy Corn Pudding 42
- Sliced Apple Cookies 43
- Chocolate Muffins 43
- Savory Spring Muffins 44
- Pita with Egg & Curry 44
- Hot Vanilla Cereals 45
- Aromatic Carrot Cream 46
- Mushrooms Velvet Soup 47
- Easy Lettuce Wraps 48
- Spaghetti with Pesto 49
- Spiced Wraps 49
- Poached Asparagus and Egg 50
- Apple Turnover 50
- Egg Drop Soup 51
- Roasted Pepper Soup 51
- Assorted Fresh Fruit Juice 52
- Raspberry and Pineapple Smoothie 53
- Mexican Frittata 53
- Olive Oil and Sesame Asparagus 54
- Breakfast Cheesecake 54
- Eggs Creamy Melt 55
- Stuffed crimini mushrooms with basil pesto 55
- DILLY SCRAMBLED EGGS with goat cheese 56
- reduced-fat BREAKFAST CASSEROLE 56
- BREAKFAST cereal mix 57
- French Toast with Tasty Strawberry Cream Cheese 57
- Cream Cheese Golden Bagel 58
- Jazz Apple oatmeal 58
- QUICK AND EASY COFFEE CUP EGG SCRAMBLE 59
- PEPPERS AND ONIONS SCRAMBLED EGG WRAP 59
- refreshing and tasty smoothie 60
- PROTEIN-PACKED TOFU SCRABLER 60
- 60-seconds omelets with veggies 61
- SAUSAGE BREAKFAST MUFFIN with EGG AND CHEESE 61
- high-protein peach smoothie 62

Tasty Breakfast Tortillas with Red Hot Jalapeno	62
Breakfast Bar with Bran and Oatmeal	63
Sweet Crepes with Apples	63
Sweet and Crunchy Popcorn	64
Fiber Booster Bars	65
Cranberry Oatmeal and Vanilla Cookies	65
Chocolate Banana Oatmeal Morning-Boost	66
Egg and Sausage Brunch	66
Stuffed Anaheim Chili Peppers	67
Puffed Tortillas Breakfast	68
Tasty Vegan Breakfast	69

LUNCH 71

Salad with Vinaigrette	72
Salad with Lemon Dressing	72
Shrimp with Salsa	73
Cauliflower Soup	74
Cabbage Stew	74
Rice and Chicken Soup	75
Herbed Chicken	76
Pesto Pork Chops	77
Vegetable Curry	77
Grilled Steak with Salsa	78
Eggplant and Red Pepper Soup	79
Persian Chicken	80
Pork Souvlaki	80
Chicken Stew	81
Baked Flounder	81
Caraway Cabbage and Rice	82
Chicken and Sweet Potato Stir Fry	82
Chicken and Asparagus Pasta	83
Hawaiian Rice	84
Shrimp Fried Rice	84
Vegetarian Egg Fried Rice	85
Autumn Orzo Salad	86
Blackened Shrimp and Pineapple Salad	86
Green Pepper Slaw	87
Cranberries and Couscous Salad	87
Tuna Salad	88
Roasted Vegetable Salad	88
Chicken Pita Pizza	89
Chicken Wraps	90
Mexican Chicken Pizza	90
Energetic Fruity Salad	91
Appealing Green Salad	91
Excellent Veggie Sandwiches	92
Lunchtime Staple Sandwiches	92
Greek Style Pita Rolls	93
Healthier Pita Veggie Rolls	93
Crunchy Veggie Wraps	94
Surprisingly Tasty Chicken Wraps	94
Authentic Shrimp Wraps	95
Loveable Tortillas	95

- Elegant Veggie Tortillas 96
- Delightful Pizza 96
- Winner Kabobs 97
- Tempting Burgers 97
- Tastiest Meatballs 98

DINNER 100

- Lemon Sprouts 101
- Lemon and Broccoli Platter 101
- Chicken Liver Stew 102
- Mushroom Cream Soup 102
- Garlic Soup 103
- Simple Lamb Chops 103
- Garlic and Butter-Flavored Cod 104
- Tilapia Broccoli Platter 104
- Parsley Scallops 105
- Blackened Chicken 105
- Spicy Paprika Lamb Chops 106
- Steamed Fish 106
- Mushroom and Olive Sirloin Steak 107
- Kale and Garlic Platter 107
- Blistered Beans and Almond 108
- Eggplant Crunchy Fries 108
- Oregano Salmon with Crunchy Crust 109
- Broiled Shrimp 109
- Shrimp Spaghetti 110
- Teriyaki Tuna 110
- Chicken Noodle Soup 111
- Beef Stew with Apple Cider 111
- Chicken Chili 112
- Tofu Stir Fry 112
- Broccoli Pancake 113
- Tangy Whole Roasted Sea Bass with Oregano 113
- Pan-Seared Salmon Salad with Lemon-Dressing 114
- Grilled Steak served with Creamy Peanut Sauce 114
- Lean Steak with Oregano-Lemon Chimichurri & Arugula Salad 115
- Herbed London Broil 116
- Ground Beef Tacos 116
- Pepper Crusted Steak 117
- Stir-Fried Chicken with Water Chestnuts 117
- Lemon Garlic Salmon 118
- Pan-Fried Chili Beef with Toasted Cashews 118
- Healthy Keto Coconut-Lime Skirt Steak 119
- Spicy Grilled Cod 120
- Healthy Low-Carb Grilled Turkey 120
- Satisfying Arugula Salad with Fruit & Chicken 121
- Tasty Coconut Cod 121

SIDES AND SNACKS 123

- Citrus Sesame Cookies 124
- Traditional Spritz Cookies 124
- Classic Baking Powder Biscuits 125
- Crunchy Chicken Salad Wraps 125
- Tasty Chicken Meatballs 126
- Herb Roasted Cauliflower 126
- Sauteed Butternut Squash 127
- German Braised Cabbage 127
- Walnut Pilaf 128
- Wild Mushroom Couscous 128
- Spicy Kale Chips 129
- Cinnamon Tortilla Chips 129
- Sweet and Spicy Kettle Corn 130
- Five-Spice Chicken Lettuce Wraps 130
- Meringue Cookies 131
- Cornbread 131
- Roasted Red Pepper and Chicken Crostini 132
- Baba Ghanoush 132
- Mixed-Grain Hot Cereal 133
- Cinnamon-Nutmeg Blueberry Muffins 133
- Fruit and Cheese Breakfast Wrap 134
- Egg-In-The-Hole 134
- Skillet-Baked Pancake 135
- Tuna Cucumber Bites 135
- Cinnamon Candied Almonds 136

FISH AND SEAFOODS ENTRÉES 138

- Grilled Shrimp with Cucumber Lime Salsa 139
- Shrimp Scampi Linguine 139
- Crab Cakes with Lime Salsa 140
- Seafood Casserole 141
- Sweet Glazed Salmon 141
- Herb-Crusted Baked Haddock 142
- Shore Lunch–Style Sole 142
- Baked Cod with Cucumber-Dill Salsa 143
- Cilantro-Lime Flounder 144
- Herb Pesto Tuna 144
- Grilled Calamari with Lemon And Herbs 145
- Lemony Haddock 145
- Glazed Salmon 146
- Tuna Casserole 146
- Oregano Salmon with Crunchy Crust 147
- Sardine Fish Cakes 147
- Cajun Catfish 148
- Poached Gennaro/Seabass with Red Peppers 148
- 4-Ingredients Salmon Fillet 149
- Oregano Grilled Calamari 149
- Baked Shrimp Crabs 150
- Salmon Stuffed Pasta 150

MEAT AND POULTRY ENTRÉES 152

- Baked Pork Chops 153
- Beef Kabobs With Pepper 153
- Cabbage and Beef Fry 154
- Mushroom and Olive Sirloin Steak 154
- California Pork Chops 155
- Beef Chorizo 155
- Pork Fajitas 156
- Caribbean Turkey Curry 156
- Chicken Fajitas 157
- Chicken Veronique 158
- London Broil 158
- Sirloin with Squash and Pineapple 159
- Slow-Cooked BBQ Beef 159
- Barley Chicken Salad 160
- Chicken Coleslaw Salad 160
- Berry-Chicken Pasta Salad 161
- Mexican-Style Chicken Salad 162
- Satay-Inspired Chicken Salad 162
- Grilled Chimichurri Chicken Kebabs 163
- Roasted Herb and Lemon Chicken with Mashed Sweet Potatoes 164
- Chicken and Broccoli Pan Bake 164
- Moroccan Chicken and Vegetable Stew 165
- Mushroom Turkey Burgers with Powerhouse Salsa 166
- Thai-Style Chicken Stir-Fry 166
- Vegetable and Turkey Kebabs 167
- Turkey Pho 167
- Turkey-Asparagus Risotto 168
- Turkey Tenderloin with Berry Sauce 169

DESSERTS 171

- Dessert Cocktail 172
- Baked Egg Custard 172
- Gumdrop Cookies 173
- Apple Crunch Pie 173
- Spiced Peaches 174
- Vanilla Custard 174
- Blueberry and Apple Crisp 175
- Lemon Mousse 175
- Raspberry Popsicle 176
- Easy Fudge 176
- Hearty Cucumber Bites 177
- Cauliflower Bagel 177
- Almond Crackers 178
- Cashew and Almond Butter 178
- Nut and Chia Mix 179
- Very Berry Bread Pudding 179
- Sunburst Lemon Bars 180
- Creamy Mint Chocolate Brownies 181
- Festive Cream Cheese Sugar Cookies 181
- Dandelion Green Smoothie 182
- Chocolate Chip Cookies 182
- Baked Peaches with Cream Cheese 183

Strawberry Ice Cream	183
Raspberry Brûlée	184

SAUCES, DRESSING AND SEASONINGS 186

Easy Garlicky Cherry Tomato Sauce	187
Roasted Onion Dip	187
Golden Turmeric Sauce	188
Creamy Turmeric Dressing	189
Dijon Mustard Vinaigrette	189
Anti-Inflammatory Caesar Dressing	190
Fresh Tomato Vinaigrette	190
Ginger Sesame Sauce	191
Golden Turmeric Tahini Sauce	191
Healthy Teriyaki Sauce	192
Yogurt Garlic Sauce	192
Chunky Tomato Sauce	193
Sweet Balsamic Dressing	193
Citrus Salad Sauce	194
Anti-Inflammatory Applesauce	194
Dried Herb Rub	195
Mediterranean Seasoning	195
Hot Curry Powder	196
Cajun Seasoning	196
Ras El Hanout	197
Poultry Seasoning	197
Adobo Seasoning Mix	198
Herbs De Provence	198
Honey Mustard	199
Pickles	199
Teriyaki Sauce	200
Alfredo Sauce	200
Tomato Salsa	201
Fajita Flavor Marinade	201
Garlic-Herb Seasoning	202
Lime Caribbean Dressing	202

Made in the USA
Middletown, DE
27 March 2023